Principles of Cardiovascular Neural Regulation in Health and Disease

BASIC SCIENCE FOR THE CARDIOLOGIST

1. B. Levy, A. Tedgui (eds.): *Biology of the Arterial Wall.* 1999
   ISBN 0-7923-8458-X
2. M.R. Sanders, J.B. Kostis (eds): *Molecular Cardiology in Clinical Practice.* 1999.   ISBN 0-7923-8602-7
3. B. Swynghedauw (ed.): *Molecular Cardiology for the Cardiologist.* Second Edition. 1998.   ISBN: 0-7923-8323-0
4. B. Ostadal, F. Kolar (eds.): *Cardiac Ischemia: From Injury to Protection.* 1999.   ISBN: 0-7923-8642-6
5. H. Schunkert, G.A.J. Riegger (eds.): *Apoptosis in Cardiac Biology.* 1999
   ISBN: 0-7923-8648-5
6. A, Malliani, (ed.): *Principles of Cardiovascular Neural Regulation in Health and Disease .* 2000.   ISBN: 0-7923-7775-3

KLUWER ACADEMIC PUBLISHERS - DORDRECHT/BOSTON/LONDON

Principles of Cardiovascular Neural Regulation in Health and Disease

by
Alberto Malliani
Professor of Internal Medicine

Centro Ricerche Cardiovascolari, CNR;
Dipartimento Scienze Precliniche LITA-Vialba;
Dipartimento di Medicina Interna, Ospedale "L. Sacco";
Università di Milano, Italy

KLUWER ACADEMIC PUBLISHERS

Boston/Dordrecht/London

Distributors for North, Central and South America:
Kluwer Academic Publishers
101 Philip Drive
Assinippi Park
Norwell, Massachusetts 02061 USA

Distributors for all other countries:
Kluwer Academic Publishers Group
Distribution Centre
Post Office Box 322
3300 AH Dordrecht, THE NETHERLANDS

Library of Congress Cataloging-in-Publication Data

Malliani, Alberto.
  Principles of cardiovascular neural regulation in health and disease/by Alberto
Malliani.
    P.; cm.--(Basic science for the cardiologist; 6)
  Includes bibliographical references and index.
  ISBN 0-7923-7775-3
    1. Cardiovascular system--Innervation. 2. Nervous system, Vasomotor. 3.
Cardiovascular system--Pathophysiology. I. Title. II. Series.
  [DNLM: 1. Cardiovascular Physiology--Cardiovascular Diseases. 2. Homeostasis--
Cardiovascular Diseases. 3. Sympathetic Nervous System--Cardiovascular diseases.
WG 102 M254p 2000]
  QP113.4.M35 2000
  612.1--dc21   00-020847

This book is dedicated to the future of my children
Davide, Anna Rachele and Eleonora and to the
courage of their grandmother Rachel Krajka.

CONTENTS

Chapter 3

Chapter 4

Chapter 5
VARIABILITY AND NONLINEAR DYNAMICS 149

Scientific *"respect for irrelevant things is increasing to gigantic proportions"*. Paraphrasing an aphorism by Karl Kraus (*Pro domo et mundo*, Vienna 1912).

PREFACE

This book is an attempt to indicate a simple way of approaching the complexity of cardiovascular neural regulation. To do so, it describes the trajectory of forty years of research, not as a personal travelogue that would be devoid of interest for most readers, but rather as a pursuit of some general principles stemming out from the complexity that I have encountered during this journey and that have determined its evolution.

A trajectory is not simply a sequence of experiments, as without adequate hypotheses the multitude of findings depicts only an irrelevant halo. Never is a trajectory the only possible one, and all hypotheses have their dialectic counterpart.

Here is where the scientific method becomes essential, being nothing else than a splendid game of intuitions and deductions in the arena of approximation. Trajectory, hypothesis, method, none of them is unique.

Admittedly, the emerging general principles often correspond to the same general hypotheses intended to be proved - and thus some subjective circling seems unavoidable.

As W.B. Cannon has lightly written (1945), *"Investigators are commonly said to be engaged in a search for the truth. I think they themselves would usually state their aims less pretentiously. What the experimenter is really trying to do is to learn whether facts can be established which will be recognized as facts by others and which will support some theory that in imagination he has projected. But he must be ingenuously honest..... The tragedy of scientific inquiry, as Huxley once remarked, is the slaying of a beautiful hypothesis by an ugly fact"*.

In this unavoidable uncertainty pertaining to the forefront of scientific reasoning, how would we detect in time the path that will eventually become an alley – to be later abandoned for a new almost invisible track? We simply cannot.

"Time past and time future allow but a little consciousness" (T.S. Eliot).

What might remain of all this endeavor is surely something different from what we expected, including nothing. We must accept that one day our conquered verities might lie at the bottom of a dry pool.

However, when an experiment is carried out carefully, with an adequate methodology and honestly described, it should enter the virtual Louvre of human accomplishments: what may change subsequently is its interpretation but not its essence.

A sound progress should be based on a conscious evaluation of all experiments which have provided the original notions. Even in the information era this is not yet feasible with a unique intelligent processor, while the scientific community tries to be a substitute. Hence, in our attempts to reach some general vision we have to rely on accounts from experts in the various fields. Thus no true objectivity can be present in what is often called the state of art. However, this scientific substrate, like any other cultural structure, presents what I would call nodal points, often corresponding to general principles: these are the crossroads where major intersections occur, where terms assume a multidisciplinary valency, where scientific debate is more essential and productive.

The scientific process is a human faculty relying on the most different attributes of our nature. Without a deep love for hypotheses no truly innovative trajectory can evolve. But this evolution requires also an ethical commitment that in this case corresponds to the capability of bearing the reality - Eliot again, "*human kind cannot bear very much reality*".

By now I cannot help thinking I am able to recognize those who truly believe in the ethics of research from those who merely utilize its economical and social benefits. The two tribes are totally different: what is perilous sailing and Mozart on one side, including the tragic event of a wrong hypothesis, becomes safe floating and heavy metal on the other.

The torch of this ethically committed research is handed down from one generation to another and so is perpetuated as one of the most precious gifts to explore our absolute need of understanding life.

So much effort spent for hypotheses may appear ridiculous and yet is a great privilege that colors the days. The point is that a hypothesis is never the final goal, but rather a formal container for a way of thinking often related to a way of being.

I have met numerous admirable researchers. Those that mostly impressed me all had in common one peculiar characteristic – their generous attempt to extract from their specific experience the sense of it and the need to express it in simple terms. It was often touching to discover that the more they proceded the simpler it was to understand the nub of their wisdom.

My attempt, now, is no presumption. It is rather a responsibility I feel, in response to the privilege of having had so much time to search.

It is also important to underline that this book is not intended to summarize the traditional knowledge on cardiovascular neural regulation which can be found in numerous and excellent books (Heymans and Neil 1958; Bishop et al. 1983; Spyer 1990; Zucker and Gilmore 1991). Conversely, it attempts to extract from such a knowledge some general points of view and to contrast them with different perspectives stemming from strictly related and more recent findings. Thus, fields of extreme relevance such as the transduction systems or the transgenic technology have not been addressed as outside the main design.

While I am writing these pages, the book is almost finished. To me it is like a novel. What will its impact on an innocent reader be? I truly don't know. But I honestly hope that some of such general principles conveyed by this book might stimulate not only researchers but also clinicians, especially if acquainted with the same principles but under a different vest. A few of such profitable intersections would already justify this endeavor.

In *Chapter 1* a conceptual pillar like *homeostasis* is contrasted with the much less appreciated and probably more frequently occurring event of *instability*. The functional properties and the reflex effects of cardiovascular sympathetic afferent fibers are under a particular scrutiny, because studying them led to the description of excitatory *positive feedback* cardiovascular reflexes. A continuous interaction of opposing mechanisms, with *negative and positive feedback* characteristics, is indeed thought to subserve the multitude of patterns pertaining to the physiological design.

In *Chapter 2* the finalistic design of physiological patterns fades out, replaced by largely purposeless and even more complex neural mechanisms such as those accompanying ischemic heart disease, arterial hypertension, congestive heart failure. These often abnormal neural mechanisms are of paramount clinical importance, indicating that both health and disease are innervated entities. An important parenthesis is opened on cardiac pain, as the most studied and relevant example of visceral pain. A peculiar *spatio/temporal pattern* is hypothesized at the basis of the nociceptive code. This hypothesis offers a plausible explanation for the elusive link between myocardial ischemia and pain, observed both in animal experiments and in the course of human disease. Thus, the traditional view that the heart possesses a sensory innervation with specific nociceptors and hence an alarm system is discarded on both experimental and clinical grounds.

In *Chapter 3* the complexity of cardiovascular neural regulation is explored in the frequency domain, by applying sophisticated but simply explained computer techniques to the assessment of cardiovascular rhythm.city. Three main black boxes are considered to participate in the genesis of cardiovascular oscillations with a period longer than cardiac cycle: *central neural integration,* peripheral inhibitory reflex mechanisms with *negative feedback* characteristics, and peripheral excitatory reflex mechanisms with *positive feedback* characteristics. This complex interaction is reflected by the state of the *sympathovagal balance* that can be indirectly assessed by using the power spectral analysis of cardiovascular variability signals such as the RR interval. This *rhythmic code* seems to provide an information that cannot be obtained with the more traditional *intensity code.*

In *Chapter 4* a necessary introductory part analyzes the characteristics and the limitations of the major tools we have to assess the disturbances of cardiovascular neural regulation in human pathophysiology. Subsequently a necessarily limited survey is attempted of some relevant pathophysiological findings that have been obtained with these new approaches. Merits and shortcomings of spectral methodology, which attempts to provide a unitary vision of complex disturbances, are progressively emerging.

In *Chapter 5* another aspect of complexity is described. Cardiovascular and in particular heart period variability – most of the times the term heart rate variability, HRV, is used in view of its widely gained acceptance – are only in part the result of rhythmical oscillations, corresponding to *linear dynamics.* In addition, *nonlinear dynamics* as well plays a role of paramount importance. The main aim has been to select examples and models that do not require particular technical knowledge to be appreciated in their biological relevance.

Throughout the whole book, as in my life, I never forget that I am also an internist. As such, although often using some reductionistic models, I do my best to remain a pupil at the school of complexity. Quite often the main task of an internist is to reassemble the disarticulated pieces, including mind, of a patient scrutinized with too specialistic and subspecialistic criteria. Despite an asymmetrical and discontinuous knowledge an internist can succeed in this task, provided he has some ability of vertical reasoning (Blois 1988) and adequate training in complexity. Such training is one of the aims of these pages.

In a sense at this point the book may be concluded. But this is where I take the liberty of adding *Chapter 6,* dealing with the principle of all principles.

Science and medicine make sense only if related to human condition and its needs. This corresponds to saying that the whole process requires an ethical structure. Thus the text attempts to define a profile of the actual state of affairs in this perspective. Avoiding any nostalgia, it is argued that the neutrality of science - if it has ever existed – is in serious danger. Too numerous and invasive emblems at the birth of this new millennium appear as quantitative Golems, whose troublesome names correspond to conflict of interest, industrial-scientific complex, progressive loss of the art of patient-physician relationship and so on, all pertaining to the alienating pursuit of an endless accumulation of wealth. Perhaps, these considerations should conclude all scientific books, thus contributing to the preservation of a human-oriented science.

The complexity of human relationships is also a determinant of this book. Probably no sentence would be the same had I not interacted with the persons that have enriched my scientific life. Hence I have to mention at least some of them.

The whole game started in Siena, where Professor Cesare Bartorelli was a gifted clinician and an extraordinarily stimulating Head. Alberto Zanchetti was still a young investigator who initiated me to the experimental method. In those years, largely spent seeking the horizon, I collaborated with Emilio Bizzi, Giancarlo Carli and with Pedro Rudomin who was visiting the laboratory. At that time no scientific project was less than a fully committed expectation. Attracted by the scientific work of Dominick P. Purpura, I went to Columbia University in New York City and there I was marked forever by the respect for complexity. Seminars around Harry Grundfest, Dom Purpura, and those in Pisa around Giuseppe Moruzzi, were also unforgettable seances of intelligence at the service of the ethics of science.

Back to Italy I went to Milan. My first team included Peter J. Schwartz, Giorgio Recordati, Massimo Pagani and Federico Lombardi, in order of age. Most of my coworkers have also been close friends in life, sharing dreams, delusions, adaptations and, of course, hypotheses. Collaborating in numerous instances with Arthur M. Brown has surely represented a splendid human and scientific experience. Vernon S. Bishop and Franco Lioy visited the laboratory in crucial moments of its development.

As time passes some coworkers take their own path, others remain raising the third generation of researchers and these the fourth one. I would so much like to mention all of them, but their names are on the papers that fully reflect the sense of this common adventure.

During the last two decades an intense collaboration with Sergio Cerutti and his coworkers at the Department of Bioengineering has played a fundamental role in the development of new experimental tools and strategies. Moreover, during the last years, our work underwent a remarkable enrichment by collaborating with Virend K. Somers, Frank M. Abboud and their coworkers in Iowa City and with David Robertson and his group in Nashville. Still in this perspective I want to thank my dear friend Bernard Swynghedauw, Pascale Mansier and their coworkers in Paris, not only for our scientific interaction but for Bernard stimulating also the birth of this book.

To close with my gratitude to scientific life, I have to write a few words about Bernard Lown, the world renowned Bostonian cardiologist. He accepted with Evgenii Chazov the 1985 Nobel Peace Prize, on behalf of the International Physicians for the Prevention of Nuclear War. He is a great scientist, a man of immense courage and a precious friend who, more than anybody else, has reinforced in me the conviction that it is at margins of medical science that the ethical role of physicians is enhanced.

Acknowledgements

I wish to express my most profound gratitude to my younger coworkers Raffaello Furlan, Stefano Guzzetti, Ornella Rimoldi, Giulia Sandrone, Laura Dalla Vecchia, Chiara Cogliati, who have offered their generous contribution to this work. Concerning the writing of this book I have to thank in particular Alberto Porta and Nicola Montano for their continuous help. Finally, all my gratitude to Isabella Ghirardelli for having provided the manuscript with a computer vest.

Chapter 1
GENERAL CONCEPTS AND HYPOTHESES IN THE STUDY OF CARDIOVASCULAR NEURAL REGULATION

Concepts are tools, useful for thinking. Hypotheses are also tools, useful for investigating.

In the field of cardiovascular neural regulation, general concepts and hypotheses are only but a few. The term *homeostasis* is the inescapable incipit.

In its intuitive terms it probably pertains to human wisdom and, as such, surely precedes the birth of experimental physiology. There is, however, a general agreement in regarding the *milieu intérieur* of Claude Bernard (1878) as the matrix of Walter Cannon's (1932) *homeostasis*. *"La fixité du milieu intérieur est la condition de la vie libre, indépendante: le mécanisme qui la permet est celui qui assure dans le milieu intérieur le maintien de toutes les conditions nécessaires à la vie des éléments"* (Bernard 1878). The sentence suggests that stability and freedom are linked as fundamental attributes of life. Stability being an obvious concept, freedom must refer to the range of worlds and activities which an organism may enter and survive (Yamamoto 1965). However, the interpretation of the relationship between stability and freedom is not so transparent: one way to achieve stability might be giving up freedom to invade certain areas or curtailing the range of activity. Moreover, the stability that appears intuitively highly desirable for intracellular or extracellular fluids cannot indiscriminately be considered as useful for other controlled variables. As is the case of arterial blood flow and pressure, the sudden changes of which are so crucial to permitting performances like strenuous exercise, fight or flight, which often ensure the very threshold for freedom, i.e. survival. In fact, Cannon's interpretation of "Wisdom of the body" (1932) largely based on homeostatic principles seems to underestimate the fact that in emergencies the sympathetic nervous system promotes the changes, rather than compensating for them (Recordati 1984). Yet, not surprisingly, Cannon wrote (1932) that *"responses of the organism itself to situations in the external environment, are associated with disturbances of the internal environment"*. Thus instability as well appears to be part of the same biological planning. In general, *homeostasis*, i.e. *stability* and its loss, i.e. *instability*, are likely to be but the extremes of a continuum spectrum.

In addition, and from another point of view, it is clear that organisms are thermodynamically open systems and that living processes are *homeodynamic* and not *homeostatic* (Rose 1998). Thus, the metaphor of homeostasis in a sense constrains our view of living systems.

An additional concept that has to be included in these basic premises is *feedback*. This term proves that along the last decades there has been a striking similarity between ideas in engineering and in the study of regulatory mechanisms in physiology. The term *"arose in the engineering context to denote a type of connectivity in which the consequences (output) of an action produced by a machine are returned in some fashion to participate in the causes (input) of the mechanical action"* (Yamamoto 1965). In the traditional biological reasoning while homeostasis implies stability, the term feedback deals with the organization of this process. That is to say that feedback mechanisms have been exclusively assigned to the biological strategy searching for *stability* (Sagawa 1983).

THE NEGATIVE FEEDBACK

When Heymans and his coworkers, at the end of the twenties, observed the hypotensive reflex elicited by increasing the arterial pressure in a recipient dog carotid sinus perfused with the blood of a donor dog, they were probably the first ones to witness the operational characteristics of a circuit with *negative feedback* characteristics (Heymans 1929). Electronic devices were still to come.

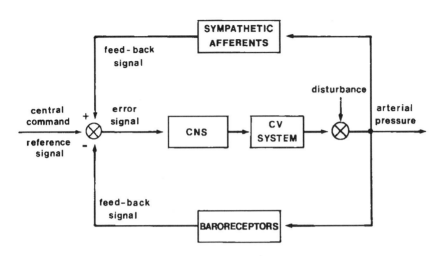

Figure 1: Schema of suggested mechanisms underlying nervous control of arterial blood pressure regulation. Baroreceptors are indicated as an example of receptors that activate negative feedback mechanisms. See text and Appendix. (From Malliani et al. 1986b, with permission).

Nowadays, a *negative feedback* circuit is usually schematized as in the inferior half of Figure 1. The schema implies that a rise in arterial pressure, by distending arterial baroreceptive areas, increases the firing activity of stretch receptors with afferent nerve fibers running in the sinus nerves and in the vagi and projecting to the medulla. The sign minus, in the scheme, indicates the inhibitory effect exerted by this afferent discharge on the neural mechanisms regulating the arterial pressure in the central nervous system (CNS): thus, the excitatory sympathetic efferent discharge directed to the cardiovascular (CV) system is reflexly decreased, while the vagal inhibitory discharge directed to the heart is reflexly increased. In broad terms, an increase in arterial pressure would induce a reflex bradycardia and a reduction in myocardial contractility and systemic vascular resistance (Spyer 1990).

In general, the common observation that arterial blood pressure in a resting man or in anesthetized animals is relatively constant and that powerful reflexes tend to counteract its changes, provided the most factual basis to the teleological concept of circulatory homeostasis. Accordingly, the sinoaortic *negative feedback* control system has been regarded for decades as the indisputable leader of this homeostasis.

On the other hand, instability has been attributed either to the overall power of the centers (the *central command* of Figure 1) or to a less efficient reflex buffering activity of negative feedback mechanisms (Sagawa 1983).

THE CENTRAL NEURAL MECHANISMS

The role played by *central mechanisms* in the regulation of sympathetic outflow was already clearly evident in the experiments on sham rage behavior by Cannon and Britton (1925) and Bard (1928). It was observed that after decortication, or brain transection sparing the posterior pole of the diencephalon, a cat is not only capable of integrated rage behavior but seems increasingly susceptible to fits of angry behavior, either spontaneously or after innocuous (e.g. tactile) stimulation. These phasic outbursts were made up of characteristic somatic phenomena, such as clawing movements, struggling, biting and a snarling expression, together with visceral phenomena, such as pupil dilatation, blood pressure increase, tachycardia and augmented respiration.

In such conditions the sympathetic outflow was likely to be activated massively as a whole; simultaneously, the parasympathetic outflow was likely to be inhibited. This was one of the initial steps towards the concept of reciprocal organization regulating the two visceral nervous outflows (Cannon 1932).

In such acute decorticate cats we demonstrated, almost forty years ago (Bizzi et al. 1961), that stimulation of the carotid body chemoreceptors (by intrasinusal injection of lobeline or administering low-oxygen mixtures) was consistently capable of evoking sham rage outbursts, identical in pattern and intensity both to outbursts induced by tactile or noxious stimulation and occurring spontaneously. Since lobeline and hypoxia ceased to evoke sham rage outbursts after selective inactivation of the carotid body chemoreceptors, it was concluded that the diencephalic mechanisms for rage behavior lie within the sphere of the excitatory influence of chemoreceptive reflexes. Conversely, the stimulation of carotid sinus baroreceptors was capable of inhibiting sham rage behavior (Bartorelli et al. 1960). Hence, peripheral stimuli acting within the cardiovascular system could influence the activity of diencephalic centers.

In those same years, an authoritative academic voice, Philip Bard (1960), asserted in the opening lecture of an international symposium that suprabulbar influences must inhibit baroreceptor function when an organism has to maintain an elevated heart rate in the face of an increased arterial pressure, as happens during periods of stress or exercise. Moruzzi (1940) had already shown that carotid sinus reflexes could be inhibited by stimulation of anterior vermis of the cerebellum. It was, however, only the subsequent progressive exploration into the hemodynamic conditions occurring during exercise or emotion (Rushmer et al. 1960; Bergamaschi and Longoni 1973; Vatner and Pagani 1976) that revealed that the negative feedback baroreflexes could change to such an extent (Bristow et al. 1971; Coote et al. 1971; Smith 1974; Vatner and Pagani 1976) that they became sometimes quite permissive bystanders in such circulatory "storms" (Lewis 1931).

As for the mechanisms through which baroreflexes could be attenuated, early attention was paid to the suprabulbar structures (Hilton 1966; Smith 1974). Subsequently it was realized that the mechanisms inhibiting the baroreflexes could be activated also from the periphery, through vagal (Vatner et al. 1975) or somatic (Kumada et al. 1975) afferent nerve fibers.

On the whole, this traditional conceptual framework included notions such as Sherrington's (1906) *dominance of the brain*, Langley's view (1903) of the sympathetic nervous system as a pure *outflow*, and the conviction that only the afferent fibers projecting directly to supraspinal structures conveyed important information from cardiovascular reflexogenic areas (Heymans and Neil 1958). *Homeostasis* and *instability* could be both explained within this neural substratum.

However, in this interpretation of cardiovascular neural regulation, an entire afferent channel, as fully described by anatomists, connecting the cardiovascular system with the central neural structures, had been completely neglected from a functional point of view. Such was the case of cardiovascular sympathetic afferent nerve fibers (Malliani 1982). The description of their functional characteristics and of their reflex effects is crucial in this attempt to extract general hypotheses, since this would lead to the notion of excitatory *positive feedback* mechanisms and to the general hypothesis of a continuous interaction of opposing mechanisms.

This section will be more detailed as this afferent channel is still largely ignored by textbooks.

THE CARDIOVASCULAR SYMPATHETIC
AFFERENT FIBERS

Edgeworth (1892) first suggested the existence of afferent nerve fibers in the cardiac sympathetic nerves which he called *sympathetic sensory fibres*. Langley (1903) also sporadically wrote about *afferent sympathetic fibres* but eventually rejected the expression with his definition of the autonomic nervous system being pure outflow. It is well known that, following Professor Jebb's suggestion, Langley (1898) coined the term *autonomic*, indicating that the structures supplied by the system are not subject to voluntary control but operate to a large extent independently. The afferent fibers in the sympathetic nerves were considered *somatic*, because they had their cell bodies in the dorsal spinal ganglia together with somatic neurons, because they were thought to have no reflex role, and because their function was assumed to be exclusively nociceptive (Langley 1903). Visceral pain also gave rise to much discussion, *"the pain of visceral and somatic disease"* being attributed, still several decades later, to *"direct stimulation of a common system of pain nerves"* (Lewis and Kellgren 1939-1942).

In short, during the same years that witnessed Sherrington's enlightening experiments leading to the coexisting concepts of *proprioceptive reflex* and *dominance of the brain* (1898, 1906), the visceral reflex spinal arc was considered either an oversimplification devoid of any functional significance or a basically wrong concept.

However, Langley must have had more doubts about *sympathetic* afferent fibers than we think. He wrote *"all that seems to me possible at present towards arranging afferent fibres into autonomic and somatic divisions is to consider as afferent fibres those which give rise to reflexes in autonomic tissues, and to consider all other afferent fibres as somatic"* (Langley 1903). The crucial fact was that Langley could only count on negative experiments: *"Such fibres ought when stimulated to produce reflexes of one sort or another even though slight. But in experiments made earlier I could not find with certainty reflex action of any kind..."* (1896). In short, I would like to suggest that it is likely that Langley had a more open mind on this topic than is generally believed.

We have firmly proposed (Malliani et al. 1973b, 1975a) the term *afferent sympathetic fibres* not only for simplicity and analogy with afferent vagal fibers, but because we consider this point essential to the concept that the visceral nervous system may have its basic functional unit in the spinal reflex arc. The *"reflex arc is the unit mechanism of the nervous system when that system is regarded in its integrative function"* (Sherrington 1906). Accordingly, the sympathetic input to the spinal cord may be as important to the regulation of the sympathetic outflow as the somatic spinal input is to the regulation of the somatic nervous outflow (Malliani et al. 1975a). In conclusion, the term reflects the original Winslow definition of sympathetic nerves as an ensemble of nerves *"bringing about the sympathies of the body"* (quoted by Langley 1915-1916), stresses their composite nature of efferent and afferent fibers and underlines the new experimental findings on sympatho-sympathetic reflexes (Malliani 1982). The term is now commonly used, but it became so in a sort of trivial way, without a true understanding of its significance (Malliani 1997). (See also the Appendix).

This afferent pathway has traditionally received scarce consideration in physiological studies not dealing primarily with the transmission of cardiac pain. Reasons for this are numerous. First, the favorable anatomical location of the vagi in the neck, compared with the intrathoracic seclusion of the cardiac sympathetic nerves, is likely to have influenced, for many years, the choice of vagal afferent fibers for the electrophysiological attempts to record impulses from cardiovascular receptors. In fact, only afferent nerve fibers with cardiovascular receptor endings, isolated from the rami communicantes or from the dorsal roots, but running through the sympathetic nerves, can be safely defined as cardiovascular sympathetic afferent fibers (Malliani 1982).

Yet, concepts more than facts often represent the true obstacle: in particular the concept that cardiovascular sympathetic afferent fibers had no physiological regulatory function (Heymans and Neil 1958).

Functional characteristics of cardiovascular sympathetic sensory endings

Brown (1967) first reported recordings of sympathetic nerve afferent multiunit activity being very low during spontaneous discharge and markedly increased during myocardial ischemia. This finding was interpreted as bearing only pathophysiological significance in the transmission of cardiac pain.

Ueda et al (1969) carried out the first detailed electrophysiological study of the impulse activity of cardiovascular sympathetic afferent fibers. The fibers were found to be responsive both to mechanical probing and to hemodynamic stimuli: however, these findings were again interpreted only as evidence that cardiac pain could be elicited mechanically.

Our hypothesis was, instead, that this afferent channel was tonically involved in the neural regulation of cardiovascular function and that, accordingly, it was conveying to the spinal cord a continuous flux of information. This was found to be the case. Under normal hemodynamic conditions, afferent sympathetic fibers, myelinated and nonmyelinated, with sensory endings located in the atria, ventricles, aorta, pulmonary veins, always displayed a spontaneous impulse activity (Malliani et al. 1973b; Malliani and Pagani 1976; Casati et al. 1979; Malliani 1979; Lombardi et al. 1981) (Figure 2).

A peculiar feature of this spontaneous discharge, independent of the location of the receptive field, was that it usually consisted of at most one action potential per cardiac cycle, each cycle being not necessarily accompanied by a nervous impulse. This is quite different from the repetitive firing per cardiac cycle of cardiovascular supraspinal afferents (Heymans and Neil 1958).

Numerous articles have reported the characteristics of the responsiveness of afferent sympathetic fibers with atrial (Malliani et al. 1973b; Uchida and Murao 1974b) and ventricular (Malliani et al. 1973b; Hess et al. 1974; Uchida et al 1974) endings to hemodynamic natural stimuli.

Sympathetic sensory endings were also found to be markedly excited during an interruption of coronary flow (Figure 3), obtained by stopping a pump-assisted perfusion of the left coronary artery, in the absence of mechanical manipulations of the heart (Brown and Malliani 1971; Malliani et al. 1973b; Lombardi et al. 1981).

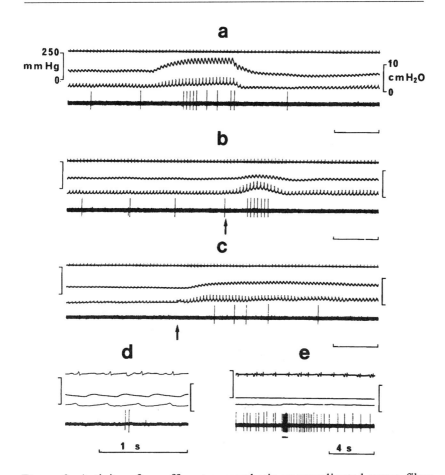

Figure 2: Activity of an afferent sympathetic nonmyelinated nerve fiber with its receptive field located in the left ventricle. Tracings represent from top to bottom, the ECG, the systemic arterial pressure, the right atrial pressure, the nervous activity (all tracings are cathode-ray oscilloscope recordings). **a** Occlusion of the descending thoracic aorta (indicated by the rise in arterial pressure); **b** i.v. injection of 5 ml warm saline, beginning at the arrow; **c** occlusion of the inferior vena cava released at the arrow; **d** electrical stimulation of the left inferior cardiac nerve activating the afferent fiber; the biphasic first deflection is the artifact of the stimulus, detectable also on the ECG trace, while the second biphasic deflection is the action potential of the fiber. The approximate length of the fiber was 3.8 cm. The conduction velocity calculated for this fiber was 0.92 m/s; **e** mechanical probing of an area of the external surface of the left ventricle, performed on the non-beating heart, after bleeding the animal to death; notice the after-discharge which is typical of group C fibers. (From Casati et al. 1979, with permission).

In the case of Figure 3, the same nonmyelinated fiber was also excited by intracoronary administration of bradykinin. In general, both myocardial ischemia and bradykinin never recruited silent afferent fibers, but only intensified the activity of spontaneously discharging units (Lombardi et al. 1981). Sometimes low doses of chemical substances appeared capable of increasing the mechanosensitivity suggesting a phenomenon of *sensitization* (Nishi et al. 1977; Lombardi et al. 1981).

Marked excitations were also obtained by simply occluding a coronary artery with a snare (Uchida and Murao 1974a; Bosnjak et al. 1979), however with the possibility of some direct mechanical stimulation of nerve fibers, even when the tract of the coronary artery to be occluded was dissected from the surrounding tissues (Casati et al 1979). As a result, various latencies for the excitatory responses were reported (Malliani 1982).

Similarly, adenosine was capable of activating the discharge of ventricular sympathetic afferent fibers and of potentiating the excitation induced by coronary occlusion (Gnecchi Ruscone et al. 1995). However, also in this case, no recruitment was ever noticed.

On the other hand, both sympathetic (Malliani et al. 1973b) and vagal (Recordati et al. 1971) myelinated afferents displayed a reduced discharge during acute hemorrhage, although this event is accompanied by a marked decrease in coronary blood flow. It is likely that the crucial difference between the two situations is represented by the size of the ventricular chambers, which is increased during acute interruption of coronary flow, but is reduced during acute bleeding.

Ventricular nonmyelinated afferents (Casati et al. 1979) do not modify their discharge during bleeding, while their impulse activity is reduced when venous return is more abruptly decreased, such as during inferior vena cava occlusion.

On the whole, these observations suggest a mechanical component in the stimulus leading to the excitation of the cardiac sensory endings during myocardial ischemia (Recordati et al. 1971; Malliani et al. 1973b)

Accordingly, I have argued (Malliani 1982) the claim by Baker et al (1980) to have identified ventricular receptors that were primarily chemosensitive, as the vast majority of data suggest a responsiveness to both mechanical and chemical stimuli.

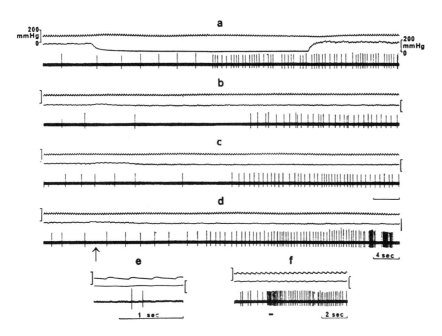

Figure 3: Activity of an afferent sympathetic nonmyelinated nerve fiber with a left ventricular sensory field.   Tracings represent, from top to bottom, systemic arterial pressure, coronary perfusion pressure, nerve impulse activity (cathode-ray oscilloscope recordings). a Interruption of the left main coronary artery perfusion; b intracoronary administration, beginning at the *arrow*, of bradykinin, 5 ng/kg; c intracoronary administration of bradykinin, 10 ng/kg; d intracoronary administration of bradykinin, 30 ng/kg; e electrical stimulation of the left inferior cardiac nerve activating the afferent fiber; the biphasic first deflection is the artifact of the fiber. The approximate length of the nerve was 8 cm. The conduction velocity calculated for this fiber was 0.45 m/s. f Mechanical probing, marked by a bar, of an area of the external surface of the left ventricle. (From Lombardi et al. 1981, with permission).

Hence, cardiac sympathetic sensory endings seem to display properties of low-threshold polymodal receptors (Burgess and Perl 1973; Malliani 1982; Malliani et al. 1989).

The mechanoceptive properties of afferent sympathetic fibers could be investigated in detail in the case of those with aortic sensory endings (Malliani and Pagani 1976). Figure 4 exemplifies such an experiment, leading to the conclusion that the receptor endings were sensitive to both the dynamic and static components of the mechanical stimulus.

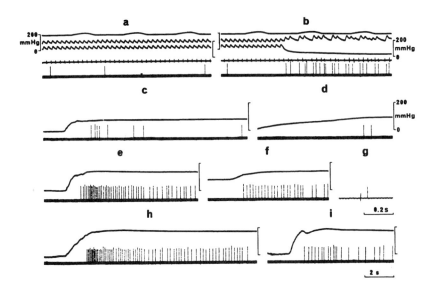

Figure 4: Activity of an afferent sympathetic nonmyelinated nerve fiber
with receptive field located in the distal third of the aortic arch. **a** Control;
b occlusion of the descending aorta; **c, d, e, f, h,** and **i**, effects of stretching
aortic wall by distending a latex balloon located in the distal part of the
aortic arch after the animal had been killed by bleeding; **g** electrical
stimulation of the left inferior cardiac nerve activating the fiber.
Approximate length of the fiber, 5 cm. Calculated conduction velocity 1
m/s. Tracings in **a** and **b** represent, from top to bottom, the endotracheal
pressure (inflations upwards), the aortic and femoral arterial pressure, the
ECG and the nervous recordings. **c, d, e, f, h,** and **i** top tracing: pressure
applied to the distending balloon; bottom tracing: nervous activity (From
Malliani and Pagani 1976, with permission).

    The pulmonary veins constitute another vascular site with a
likely reflexogenic role of paramount importance. Nonidez (1941)
observed that the pulmonary veins of previously sympathectomized
cats contained no receptor endings. In his opinion this indicated that
the sensory fibers innervating these vessels run in the sympathetic
nerves. This suggestion was confirmed by Lombardi and coworkers
(1976) who identified the impulse activity of afferent sympathetic
myelinated nerve fibers which had their endings on the pulmonary
veins. The fibers displayed a spontaneous discharge that was
remarkably sensitive to increases in pressure in the left atrium and,

consequently, in the pulmonary veins, such as those obtained with i.v. injection of warm saline or with pressor drugs. Conversely, impulse activity decreased during reductions in pulmonary venous pressure, however produced. These receptors appear particularly suitable to sense pulmonary congestion.

In conclusion, actual knowledge of cardiovascular sympathetic afferents indicates that their functional properties are very complex. In the presence of adequate hemodynamic conditions they display a spontaneous impulse activity. Some of these afferents have a single and very restricted receptive field (Malliani et al. 1973b), while others have either a large one or more than one receptive field (Malliani et al. 1973b; Coleridge et al. 1975; Malliani and Pagani 1976). It is an interesting possibility that fibers with large or multiple receptive fields might be particularly suited to signal generalized hemodynamic events such as arterial hypertension or venous congestion.

Reflex effects mediated by cardiovascular sympathetic afferent fibers

The study of the reflex effects elicited by the stimulation of cardiovascular sympathetic afferent fibers has probably contributed to the appreciation of the importance of this afferent pathway more than the detailed analysis of the functional characteristics of its receptors. In fact, it has become progressively clearer that these afferent fibers constitute by no means a kind of redundant and less sophisticated channel of information, but that instead they mediate reflexes, mainly excitatory, which are quite different from those subserved by the supraspinal cardiovascular afferent fibers.

Acute experiments

From a historical point of view, there was little in the literature to indicate that an excitatory reflex could be elicited from the cardiovascular system through an afferent sympathetic limb.

In 1940, De Waele and Van de Velde (1940) made the unexpected observation that a mechanical manipulation of the heart could produce a hypertensive response which was probably reflex in nature as its afferent limb could be interrupted by sectioning the higher thoracic dorsal roots. Subsequently, Taquini and Aviado (1961) found that a partial occlusion of the pulmonary artery could increase pulmonary blood flow. The increased flow was present after vagotomy and in spinal animals and appeared to depend on intact sympathetic innervation.

To the best of my knowledge this was the scanty experimental evidence preceding our own experiments that began with the observation that coronary occlusion could reflexly alter the firing frequency, most often toward excitation, of preganglionic sympathetic efferent fibers (Malliani et al. 1969). Recordings were obtained from single fibers isolated from the left third thoracic ramus communicans (T3), which is known to contribute to the innervation of the heart (Bronk et al. 1936; Randall et al. 1957). As the reflex response was present in animals with the vagi and spinal cord cut, a cardiocardiac spinal sympathetic reflex was proposed, the afferent and efferent pathways of which were both in the sympathetic nerves. The reflex was also present in animals with intact neuraxis and after chronic sino-aortic denervation (Figure 5).

The existence of this reflex in the dog has been denied by Felder and Thames (1979) reporting only depressor reflexes, as previously described (Costantin 1963). Their conceptual position was that *"inhibitory cardiac receptors with vagal afferents may serve a protective role by limiting increases in cardiac sympathetic nerve activity during myocardial ischemia"* (Felder and Thames 1979). As a reply I criticized their experimental preparation, consisting of acute sino-aortic denervated dogs with a very high background sympathetic activity difficult to be further incremented (Malliani 1980). However the matter was definitely settled when Minisi and Thames (1991) also reported the observation of sympathetic excitatory reflex responses elicited by transmural myocardial ischemia and mediated by cardiac sympathetic afferents.

The finding of a cardiocardiac sympathetic reflex raised the more general problem of whether natural hemodynamic events could also elicit sympathetic reflexes in spinal animals.

Numerous reports, starting with Sherrington's observations (1906), indicated the existence of vasomotor and sympathetic responses in experimental spinal animals (Langley 1924; Brooks 1933, 1935; Heymans et al. 1936; Alexander 1945; Downman and McSwiney 1946; Beacham and Perl 1964; Franz et al. 1966; Beacham and Kunze 1969) and in paraplegic man (Guttman and Whitteridge 1947). However, in spite of these descriptions it was not generally appreciated that spinal sympathetic centers may react reflexly in response to natural events, such as changes in blood pressure.

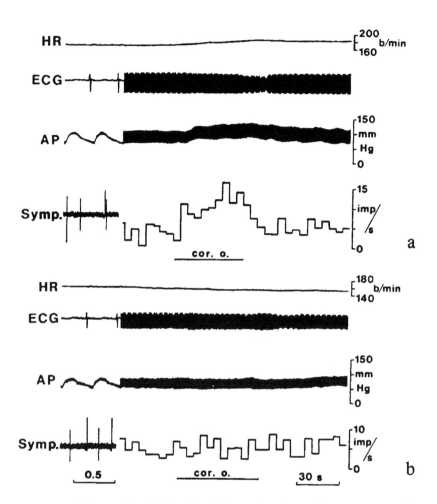

Figure 5: Effects of occluding the left anterior descending coronary artery in a vagotomized cat. Sino-aortic denervation had been performed 1 week before. Between **a** and **b** the left stellate ganglion and the left thoracic sympathetic chain were removed down to T4, thus producing a partial "sympathetic deafferentation" that, however, was sufficient for the interruption of the afferent limb of the reflex. Tracings from top to bottom are the heart rate, the ECG, the arterial pressure, the impulse activity recorded from a multifiber preparation obtained from the left T3. (From Malliani 1982, with permission).

The only suggestions for the existence of spinal vasomotor and sympathetic reflexes elicited by arterial pressure changes were to be found in accounts by Heymans et al. (1936) and by Fernandez de Molina and Perl (1965); however, in both studies the reflex nature of these responses was not properly defined.

In our experiments on spinal vagotomized cats (Malliani et al. 1971) we found that increases in systemic arterial pressure induced reflex changes in the impulse activity of single preganglionic sympathetic fibers in T3 which was either increased or decreased. The type of response was consistent for each individual fiber and was always reflex in nature. The observation that in some cases blood pressure rises as small as 15-20 mmHg elicited these reflex responses appeared to us quite remarkable, suggesting a physiological role for these spinal mechanisms (Malliani et al. 1971). When, however, the increases in pressure were restricted to the coronary circulation, by augmenting the flow of a perfusing pump, the preganglionic and postganglionic sympathetic discharge to the heart was always excited (Malliani and Brown 1970; Brown and Malliani 1971).

We subsequently designed a series of experiments (Pagani et al. 1974) in order to analyze specifically the excitatory and inhibitory components of spinal reflexes. Small rubber balloons mounted on catheters were inserted into the thoracic portions of the inferior vena cava and of the aorta, and in the infundibular region of the left ventricle. These balloons could be inflated to obstruct blood flow. In addition, the pulmonary artery or the aorta could be constricted by using snares. It was found that when the stimuli were applied to the heart, thus eliciting possible cardiocardiac reflexes, an excitatory response was the rule. Conversely, when the stimuli simultaneously affected cardiac and vascular receptors such as during rises in arterial pressure, the discharge of the same fibers was either increased or decreased.

We devised a special cannula consisting of a stainless steel tube surrounded by an inflatable rubber cylinder in order to stretch the walls of the thoracic aorta without interfering with aortic blood flow (Figure 6). In this manner it was possible to excite selectively aortic mechanoreceptors with a physical stimulus the effect of which on aortic walls was the same as an increase in mean aortic pressure. The reflex responses of each preganglionic sympathetic neuron were either excitatory or inhibitory and they were consistent and in the same direction as observed during the increases in systemic arterial pressure. It was thus obvious that receptors located in various cardiovascular sites could exert different reflex effects on the same sympathetic preganglionic neuron.

We therefore advanced the hypothesis that a prevalence of excitatory mechanisms existed in sympatho-sympathetic reflexes in which input and output were circumscribed to a few spinal segments, as in the case of cardiocardiac reflexes, while inhibitory mechanisms were also present in the reflexes involving more spinal segments, as during aorto-cardiac reflexes.

The reciprocal reflex action exerted by sympathetic and vagal afferents was directly investigated in experiments in which single sympathetic and vagal efferent fibers were isolated from the same cardiac nerve at its junction with the right atrium (Schwartz et al. 1973). It was found (Figure 7) that electrical or chemical stimulation of afferent cardiac sympathetic fibers elicited an excitation of sympathetic efferent fibers and a simultaneous inhibition of vagal efferent fibers.

The possibility of a synergistic effect was obvious and thus we concluded that cardiac sympathetic afferents can mediate an integrated excitatory reflex directed back to the heart. The sympathovagal component of this reflex represented a total overturning of the traditional vagosympathetic circuit.

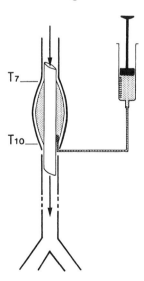

Figure 6: Schema of a cannula, consisting of a stainless steel tube surrounded by an inflatable rubber cylinder, used to stretch the walls of the thoracic aorta without interfering with aortic blood flow (From Malliani 1982, with permission).

In the same experiments, the stimulation of vagal afferents produced specular effects by exciting the vagal and inhibiting the sympathetic efferent fibers. In this case we concluded that vagal afferents can mediate an integrated inhibitory reflex directed to the heart.

Peterson and Brown (1971) were the first to assess the functional significance of reflexes mediated by sympathetic afferent fibers: they found a reflex increase in arterial pressure elicited by electrical stimulation of afferent cardiac sympathetic fibers. Subsequently it was found that similar electrical stimulations reflexly induced an increase in myocardial contractility (Malliani et al. 1972), heart rate (Malliani et al. 1973a), and aortic smooth muscle tone (Pagani et al. 1975).

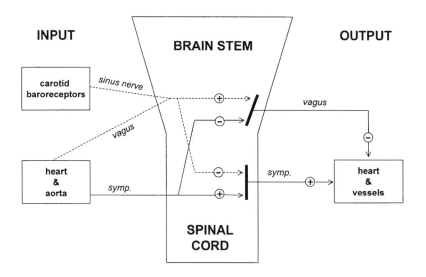

Figure 7: Schema of the neural pathways regulating from the heart and arterial baroreceptors the sympathetic and vagal activities directed to the heart (From Malliani 1997, with permission).

In particular, when the increases in myocardial contractility could be induced with intracoronary injections of veratridine (Malliani et al. 1972), conclusive evidence was obtained on the existence of a cardiocardiac sympathosympathetic reflex.

Staszewska-Barczak et al (1976), on the other hand, were able to demonstrate clearly the existence of excitatory cardiovascular reflexes elicited by the epicardial application of bradykinin and mediated by cardiac sympathetic afferent fibers.

However, it still had to be proven that cardiovascular reflex responses could be elicited by natural stimulation of sympathetic mechanoreceptors. The observation that numerous sympathetic sensory endings could be identified in the walls of the thoracic aorta by their function and that a stretch localized to a segment of it could reflexly modify the activity of sympathetic preganglionic neurons (Pagani et al. 1974), seemed to offer a possible solution to this problem. A similar aortic cannula (Figure 6) was used: in spinal vagotomized cats or in cats with an intact central nervous system but with sino-aortic denervation, stretching the thoracic aorta, which did not interfere with aortic blood flow, induced significant increases in arterial blood pressure, heart rate, and maximum rate of rise in left ventricular pressure (Lioy et al. 1974). These responses were eliminated by appropriate pharmacological blockade and by infiltrating the wall of the thoracic aorta with xylocaine.

This experiment fully demonstrated that afferent sympathetic nerve fibers can mediate excitatory cardiovascular reflexes. However, as to their physiological significance, we had to admit that most responses were obtained in anesthetized animals in which the buffering influences exerted by vagal and carotid sinus afferents had been eliminated. It was totally unproven whether such reflexes could exist in the fully innervated animal and whether a substantial activation of the cardiovascular sympathetic afferent fibers could occur in the conscious state in the absence of pain.

Chronic experiments

In order to achieve some perspective on the natural role of excitatory reflexes there was a need for models that could reveal, in the unanesthetized state and possibly in the presence of an intact innervation, functioning cardiovascular reflexes mediated by sympathetic afferent fibers.

The first model (Fig. 8) consisted of cats with a chronic spinal section performed at the level of the eighth cervical segment, breathing spontaneously, and with normal arterial pressure (Bishop

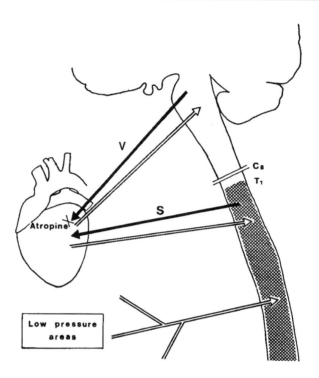

Figure 8: Schema of the animal model used in the experiments by Bishop et al (1976). A chronic spinal section was performed at the level of the eight cervical segment; atropine was administered to block the vagal outflow. The cardiac innervation with a possible reflex function was thus restricted to a sympathosympathetic loop. (From Malliani 1982, with permission).

et al. 1976). In these animals the cardiac innervation consisted of two independent loops, one vagovagal and one sympathosympathetic. Atropine (0.5-0.7 mg/kg) was administered i.v. to block the outflow of the vagal loop. Due to the chronic spinal section, the sympathetic efferent tonic activity was presumably low as suggested by the mean baseline heart rate – 109 beats/min and, after atropine, 127 beats/min. Under these conditions, i.v. infusion (Figure 9) of saline (50-150 ml) over a period of 2-5 min resulted in a significant tachycardia: the maximal increase observed was 22 beats/min, while the average was 10 beats/min. A section of thoracic dorsal roots T 1-6 and of the spinal cord between T6 and T7 abolished the response, thus proving that it was reflexly mediated through sympathetic afferent fibers.

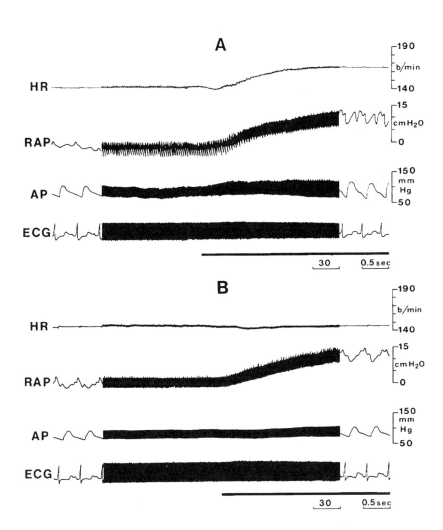

Figure 9: Analogue recording of heart rate (HR), right atrial pressure (RAP), arterial pressure (AP), and electrocardiogram (ECG) in a chronic spinal cat in control conditions and during i.v. infusions. (A) sham preparation (dorsal roots T_1-T_6 isolated but not cut); B Recordings were obtained 36 h after section of dorsal roots T_1- T_6 and of spinal cord between T_6 and T_7. Infusions indicated by bars. (From Bishop et al. 1976, with permission).

A tachycardia evoked by i.v. infusions and thought to be reflexly mediated by sympathetic afferent fibers, has also been described in anesthetized dogs (Gupta 1975; Gupta and Singh 1977).

Thus the increase in heart rate following intravenous infusions first described by Bainbridge (1915) appears to be mediated, at least partly, by afferent sympathetic fibers. Such a reflex mechanism may play an important role in the course of congestive heart failure.

The second model consisted in repeating the experiments of stretching a short segment of the thoracic aorta in conscious dogs with an intact cardiovascular innervation. In the initial experiments (Malliani et al. 1979) a metal cannula covered by a rubber cylinder, similar to that used in acute experiments (Figure 6), was implanted.

Subsequently (Pagani et al. 1982) a Teflon stiff core was employed for the cannula which allowed the use of an ultrasound technique using piezoelectric crystals to measure the external aortic diameter, in the tract surrounding the cannula, during control conditions and during the stretch. Catheters for pressure recordings, piezoelectric crystals, and the aortic cannula were all implanted under general anesthesia and aseptic conditions.

After recovery from surgery, aortic diameter was increased 9.6% ± 0.4% from 16±1 mm by inflating the implanted cannula. This stretch, which did not evoke behavioral changes produced a rise in mean aortic pressure of 31% ± 3% from 100±3 mmHg and an increase in heart rate of 20% ± 3% from 91±3 beats/min ($P<0.01$) (Pagani et al. 1982).

An example of these pressor reflexes is shown in Figure 10. Once a threshold level was exceeded, progressive increases in arterial blood pressure were obtained by augmenting distension. Alpha-adrenergic receptor blockade abolished the arterial pressure response (Fig. 10). The reflex tachycardia was prevented by combined muscarinic and β-adrenergic receptor blockade. The reflex nature of the response was, therefore, proved. As to the entity of the stimulus, some further considerations seem appropriate. First, the distension was applied to a limited portion of the thoracic aorta, corresponding to about two intercostal spaces. Secondly, a steady stimulus was used while sympathetic aortic afferents are more sensitive to pulsatile stretch (Malliani and Pagani 1976). Therefore, the activation of the mechanoreceptors of the thoracic aorta was likely to be far from maximal.

The possibility that this sympathetic reflex might interact with baroreceptor mechanisms was also investigated, because such an interplay was suggested by a previous electrophysiological study (Schwartz et al. 1973).

The slope of the regression of the electrocardiographic RR interval on the systolic pressure increase induced by phenylephrine was used as an index of baroreceptor sensitivity (Smyth et al. 1969). Aortic stretch produced a significant reduction in baroreflex sensitivity (57% ± 7 from 18±2 ms/mmHg, P<0,01). Additionally, the arterial pressure response increased after carotid nerve section and vagotomy to 49% ± 8% (Pagani et al. 1982). This observation not only confirmed that the afferent limb of the reflex was in the sympathetic nerves, but also indicated that the baroreceptive and vagal afferent fibers were likely to play a restraining role.

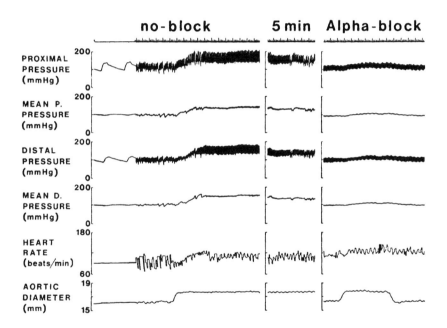

Figure 10: Pressor and heart rate responses to stretch of the descending thoracic aorta in a conscious dog. The initiation of aortic stretch (left panel) is indicated by the increase in aortic diameter. Notice the similar increase in both proximal and distal pressures, indicating the lack of direct mechanical obstruction to blood flow by aortic distension. After 5 min (middle panel), the pressure and heart rate responses were still maintained. Alfa-adrenergic blockade (phentolamine 1 mg/kg) (right panel) virtually abolishes the pressor response to aortic stretch, while an increase in heart rate is still present (From Pagani et al. 1982, with permission).

In the third model (Pagani et al. 1985b), we resorted to the intracoronary administration of bradykinin in the conscious dog. As described above, bradykinin produces marked activation of cardiac sympathetic afferent fibers (Uchida and Murao 1974c; Nishi et al. 1977; Baker et al. 1980; Lombardi et al. 1981) and in addition it substantially excites afferent cardiac vagal nonmyelinated fibers (Kaufman et al. 1980). Catheters were inserted in the aorta and either the left circumflex or anterior descending coronary artery. Bradykinin (100 ng/kg) injected into the cannulated coronary artery, 1-2 weeks after surgery, induced in the conscious animals a significant (p<0.001) increase in mean arterial pressure (28±3% from 89±4 mmHg), heart rate (30±4% from 88±beats/min), left ventricular pressure and its rate of rise (18±3% from 2812±65 mmHg/sec). Graded doses of bradykinin produced graded effects. These changes were obtained in the absence of behavioral changes suggesting a painful stimulus. The reflex nature of the various components of the response was proved by their disappearance after appropriate pharmacological blockades.

In other studies on anesthetized animals, the intracoronary administration of bradykinin produced depressor (Neto et al. 1974) or either pressor or depressor reflexes (Reinmann and Weaver 1980; Lombardi et al. 1982), the depressor component being mediated by vagal afferent fibers.

These facts clearly indicate the fundamental role played by anesthesia, when several neural circuits are simultaneously activated, in determining the final response.

In general, at difference from what suggested by experiments using a non physiological substance like veratridine in anesthetized (Von Bezold and Hirt 1867) and unanesthetized animals (Barron and Bishop 1982), the notion seems no longer tenable that a chemical stimulus applied to the neurally intact heart always elicits a vagally mediated depressor response and that vagotomy is necessary (Coleridge and Coleridge 1979) to reveal pressor sympathetic reflexes. In the conscious state, it can rather be concluded that excitatory reflexes mediated by sympathetic afferent fibers predominate during a massive stimulation of the whole cardiac sensory apparatus.

THE POSITIVE FEEDBACK

It is quite obvious that the stretch of the thoracic aorta can induce reflex changes opposite to those that would be obtained by stretching a carotid sinus. Thus, the existence of *positive feedback* mechanisms was postulated (Lioy et al. 1974; Malliani 1982; Pagani et al. 1982; Bishop et al. 1983; Malliani et al. 1986b). However, while the *negative feedback* mechanism has met an unconditioned acceptance, the proposal of a mechanism apparently devoid of any finalistic purpose has received scarce attention.

The following issues should be considered before deciding whether this reluctance might correspond to common sense or myopia.

In our view *positive feedback* reflexes are tonically operative in normal conditions for two reasons: first, aortic sympathetic mechanoreceptors generate a spontaneous impulse activity at normal arterial pressures (Malliani and Pagani 1976); secondly, the amount of aortic stretch required to elicit a pressor reflex is comparable to that accompanying rises in arterial pressure within the physiological range (Pagani et al. 1979, 1982). Similar considerations apply to sympathetic sensory endings located in the heart or vascular low pressure areas (Malliani 1982) and hence to the excitatory reflex mechanisms originating therefrom.

However, by the Darwinian hypothesis of no less value in physiology than in morphology, every reflex must be purposive. But the assignment of a specific purpose to a particular reflex is often difficult and hazardous (Woodworth and Sherrington 1904).

The *positive feedback* reflexes should be considered as one component of those complex regulatory mechanisms which result from the interplay of multiple and independent peripheral loops and of multifarious possibilities of central integration. In the resting or anesthetized state, the supraspinal structures are likely to exert a restraining influence on these reflexes (Lioy and Szeto 1975; Pagani et al. 1982). It should also be kept in mind that reflexes mediated by sympathetic afferent fibers possess inhibitory components as well (Pagani et al. 1974). In brief, the *negative feedback* mechanisms frequently seem to act as the effective controllers of the overall cardiovascular regulation. However, even in these cases, *positive feedback* mechanisms could play a regulatory role in modulating the range of operation, gain and stability of supraspinal cardiovascular reflexes. In this regard, it should be recalled that the sensitivity of *negative feedback* baroreceptive control of heart rate could be markedly reduced during aortic stretch (Malliani et al. 1979; Pagani et al. 1982). Thus, in resting conditions *positive feedback* reflexes may behave discreetly while participating in the fine tuning of homeostasis.

On the other hand, there are physiological conditions, such as exercise or emotion, in which the efferent sympathetic activity seems to be unrestricted. If a reflex must be purposive, an animal running away from a predator would find *positive feedback* mechanisms quite well suited for its goal.

In tetraplegic patients, cardiovascular sympathetic reflexes seem often to possess a savage power (Corbett et al. 1971a,b), which perhaps indicates the full potential of the system. In this context, it appears almost unthinkable that *positive feedback* sympathetic mechanisms are not even considered (Mathias and Frankel 1988) in order to explain the *autonomic dysreflexia* characterizing patients with complete quadriplegia.

"The phenomena of disease are thought to be purely adventitious; they are spoken of as 'pathological', and are supposed to bear no relation, even remotely, to any mode of response which has previously existed in the individual or the race". "Normally...(the more primitive responses) are suppressed because they would disturb the more discriminative response of higher centers; but they still remain capable of revival under conditions demanding urgent and impulsive action" (Head 1921).

THE CONTINUOUS INTERACTION OF OPPOSING MECHANISMS

What I suggest is that *negative* and *positive feedback* mechanisms interact continuously, to achieve the most adequate neural regulation of cardiovascular performance: if this were the case each specific hemodynamic condition, even one corresponding to the most stable resting state, would reflect some degree of interaction of opposite tendencies (Figure 1).

In *closed loop* conditions (Sagawa 1983) natural hemodynamic events are quite unlikely to influence the activity of one single reflexogenic area. As the mechanical threshold of sensory endings of cardiovascular sympathetic afferents seems totally comparable to that of cardiovascular supraspinal afferents (Bishop et al. 1983), it is implicit that each hemodynamic event should simultaneously activate both spinal and supraspinal afferent pathways.

However, the traditional reductionistic approach has brought the artificial fragmentation of the whole regulatory network into a legion of presumed simple reflexes and to the subsequent attempt to reconstitute a unitary vision from a collage of fragments. Although we have surely enriched our knowledge along this path, the danger of overlooking some obvious shortcomings has become also quite clear. For instance, when reconsidering the words of Sherrington (1906) *"a simple reflex is probably a purely abstract conception, because all parts of the nervous system are connected together ... and it is a system certainly never absolutely at rest"* we cannot help realizing that this caution arisen from the analysis of simple somatic reflexes has surprisingly disappeared from a field, the neural control of circulation, which has to be envisaged as a *closed loop system*.

A typical example of this way of reasoning is furnished by the usual interpretation of baroreflexes as if they were simple reflexes originated only from a restricted although bilateral reflexogenic area. Conversely it has been demonstrated, still within the traditional view of unopposed *negative f*eedback mechanisms, that multiple reflexes of the same sign (Sagawa 1983) contribute to what is called the baroreflex. In addition, however, we obtained indisputable experimental evidence that reflexes of opposite sign also contribute to the composite baroreflex integrated response.

Experiments were carried out (Gnecchi Ruscone et al. 1987) on anesthetized and decerebrate cats. A reflex bradycardia was induced by arterial pressure rises obtained either with occlusions of the thoracic aorta or with phenylephrine injections. This reflex response was significantly increased by sectioning the spinal dorsal roots from C8 to T6, causing the interruption of a large contingent of cardiovascular sympathetic afferent fibers. For instance, in decerebrate cats, the bradycardia response increased from 21±4 to 34±4% after dorsal root section.

The observation that after the rhizotomy similar arterial pressure rises were accompanied by greater reductions in heart rate was interpreted as the result of the interruption of the excitatory influences mediated by the activation of cardiovascular sympathetic afferent fibers, thus allowing a greater expression of the inhibitory baroreceptive supraspinal mechanisms. This reflex action of sympathetic afferents could consist in an excitation of the sympathetic output to the heart and/or in an increased restraint exerted on vagal efferent activity (Figure 7).

This general hypothesis, furthermore, seems to explain quite well the composite patterns characterizing the beat-to-beat spontaneous fluctuations of heart period and arterial pressure. In their original approach Bertinieri et al (1988), attempting to assess the spontaneous baroreflex, identified in the case of about one-fourth of the total number of cardiac cycles, sequences of three or more consecutive beats during which heart period and arterial pressure underwent simultaneous increases or decreases. These spontaneous episodes of hypertension/bradycardia and hypotension/tachycardia appeared to reflect baroreflex mechanisms, as they were drastically reduced by sino-aortic deafferentation. More recently, however, Legramante et al (1999) sharply observed that for about five per cent of cardiac cycles a different pattern of sequences could be identified, consisting in increases in arterial pressure and decreases in heart period or, conversely, decreases in arterial pressure and increases in heart period. These Authors hypothesized that these spontaneous episodes of hypertension/tachycardia or hypotension/bradycardia were likely to reflect the *positive feedback* mechanisms normally interacting with those of opposite sign.

As this approach cannot extract the information content embedded in each cardiac cycle but can only detect the patterns exhibited by several consecutive beats, it is impossible to extrapolate which is the prevailing mechanism operating along the remaining seventy per cent of heart beats. However, it is an appealing hypothesis that it is this continuous interaction of opposing mechanisms, with their central and peripheral reflex components, that in fact is responsible for making a given predominant pattern detectable in only about one-third of cardiac revolutions.

CONCLUSIONS

In this Chapter we have encountered such terms as *homeostasis, instability, negative and positive feedback.* Each of them corresponds to a concept-hypothesis and is, *per se,* a black box.

They all converge into a concept of *interaction* which is at the basis of complex systems. The difference existing between complex and complicated systems is well-known. A complicated system, like a watch, requires to be disassembled in order to be better understood and its total complicacy corresponds to the sum of its parts. The interactions occurring in complex systems are never linear and cannot be fragmented into pieces. When we do so we might only obtain an experimental model which is, however, a simplified version of reality. Accordingly, the total complexity is much more than the sum of its artificial subdivisions.

As to the interaction of opposite mechanisms, human culture has furnished even too strong proposals, from light and darkness in Manichaean conception to Yin and Yang in Chinese philosophy. In biology, every crucial variable seems to be under the control of opposite mechanisms. To take just an example, we now know as many factors opposing rather than favoring coagulation. Thus we are closer to understand why a clotting process can be discrete and purposeful and how the many different aspects of pathophysiology might arise.

Along this way of reasoning, it was in my opinion a great ingenuity to have assigned the neural regulation of cardiovascular function exclusively to *negative feedback* mechanisms. More thoughtfully Yamamoto (1965) has written, on pure theoretical grounds: *"Yet it should be noted that in complex systems which show a stability it is sometimes desirable or even essential to have portions of the system operate in the positive feedback mode".* This should be even more true for cardiovascular neural regulation, that knows stability only in theoretical terms, while a continuous interaction of *stability* and *instability* is more likely to fit with common observations.

Local vasomotor control, which will not be analyzed in this book, includes an endothelium derived relaxing factor (EDRF) (Furchgott and Zawadzki 1980), now identified with NO (Ignarro et al. 1987; Palmer et al. 1987), an endothelium derived contracting factor (EDCF) (Hickey et al 1985), now identified with the peptide endothelin (Yanagisawa et al. 1988), catecholamines and neuropeptide Y (Daly et al. 1987) as sympathetic modulators, and a number of additional substances. In a Lancet Review (Anonymous 1988) whose title was "Yin and Yang in vasomotor control", it was written: *"Flow-dependent dilatation and pressure-dependent constriction can be regarded as opposing positive-feedback mechanisms, each of which alone is theoretically unstable. Together with metabolic mechanisms of vasoregulation they may stabilise vasomotor tone while preserving flexibility in dynamic control"*.

This is to say that biology is the very place for dialectics.

In *Leben des Galilei* Bertolt Brecht has written: *" the aim of science is not to open a door to infinite wisdom but to set a limit to infinite error "*.

Chapter 2
PATHOPHYSIOLOGICAL MECHANISMS AND THE LOSS OF A FINALISTIC PURPOSE

Reading physiology independently of its finalistic structure should be considered almost unthinkable. On the other hand, the alteration of this finalistic organization introduces the concept of pathophysiology in the neural regulatory mechanisms. Yet it is worth noting how often the perusal of some benefit for the whole organism, in most pathophysiological regulatory mechanisms accompanying a disease or creating *per se* a disturbance, has been attempted.

To provide an example, Cyon and Ludwig (1866) had the first idea of a reflex regulation of the cardiovascular system, exercised via afferent nerve endings located in the heart and blood vessels. They found that the stimulation of the central end of the depressor nerve in the neck of the rabbit caused marked bradycardia and systemic hypotension. They believed that the depressor nerve arose from endings in the heart itself and considered that these sensory endings were normally responsive to changes in intracardiac pressure. If the heart had to beat too strongly, they concluded, the reflex bradycardia and systemic hypotension would reduce its work. That was an amazing intuition, anticipating the concept of *negative feedback* mechanism, although we know now that the aortic-depressor nerve endings are located in the aortic arch and in the roots of the great vessels (Heymans and Neil 1958).

Given this physiological framework, however, the hypothesis already mentioned (Felder and Thames 1979) – that depressor reflexes might exert a protective role in the course of acute myocardial infarction – may be misleading considering, as is reported below, that in this acute pathophysiological set excessive bradycardia is likely to be associated to an increased occurrence of sudden death.

Another crucial point is that, at least in the field of neural regulation, pathophysiological mechanisms mainly deal with abnormal quantities rather than qualities, thus generating a quantitative disturbance of regulation.

This debate, or a similar one, is in fact quite old and important if the sentence by the philosopher Auguste Comte (1828) holds true - *"Pour bien comprendre une Science il faut en connaître l'histoire"*.

Indeed defining the state of disease has always been a major challenge for human understanding. Medicine, traditionally based on pathology, has been standing for a long time on two main pillars: the concepts of cellular (Virchow) and organ (Morgagni) diseases. The resulting conception of pathological inevitably implied a different *quality* between normal and pathological. And indeed it could be so and quite often. However, as will be seen, there are processes which are better analyzed in terms of *disease of regulation* (Page 1949), to use an expression referring to arterial hypertension, a state which Pickering (1978) considered simply as an abnormal *quantity*.

In this context, it is not a question of defining *quality* and *quantity*, a hard epistemological task. The point instead is to realize, in simple biological terms, that a *disturbance of regulation* hypothesizes a continuum of quantities along a spectrum paralleled by a continuum of risk factors, its price being the disease.

In science we are deeply interested in the birth of new ideas. Mainly because science, at least biological science, has to do more with opinions than with certainties. Yet, it is much easier to assess when a fact occurs rather than when a new idea is conceived: indeed a new idea, before reaching the critical mass for its definition, is often preceded by a pre-idea, a stage which can last a long time.

Specific examples for the conception of pathological as an abnormal quantity, could be the following thoughts. Auguste Comte in his *Examen du traité de Broussais sur l'irritation* (1828) wrote: *"Partant de la grande vérité générale entrevue par Brown, que la vie ne s'entretient que par l'excitation, vérité que M. Broussais s'est rendue propre par l'important usage qu'il en a fait, il représente toutes les maladies comme consistant essentiellement dans l'excès ou le défaut de l'excitation des divers tissus, au-dessus ou au-dessous du degré qui constitue l'état normal."*

About fifty years later, Claude Bernard in his *Leçons sur la chaleur animale* (1876) wrote: *"La santé et la maladie ne sont pas deux modes différant essentiellement comme ont pu le croire les anciens médicins, et comme le croient encore quelques praticiens. Il ne faut pas en faire des principes distincts, des entités qui se disputent l'organisme vivant et qui en font le théâtre de leur lutte. Ce sont là des vieilleries médicales. Dans la réalité, il n'y a entre ces deux manières d'être que des différences de degré: l'exagération, la disproportion, la désharmonie des phénomènes normaux, constituent l'état maladif. Il n'y a pas un cas où la maladie aurait fait apparaître des conditions nouvelles, un changement complet de scène, des produits nouveaux et spéciaux."*

This was probably more than a pre-idea. And indeed, this was the basis for Bernard's experimental medicine, a holistic attempt to conceptualize normal and abnormal and a concrete way for the investigator to link experimental and clinical observations.

The neural mechanisms involved in the cardiovascular regulation are likely to be not only a link between normal and abnormal but also a solid ground for the novel certainty that health and disease are both innervated entities.

ISCHEMIC HEART DISEASE

Neural mechanisms accompanying acute myocardial infarction.

The clinical work by Pantridge's group offered a new perspective and represented a milestone (Webb et al. 1972; Pantridge 1978). As more deaths from acute myocardial infarction occur within one hour from the onset of symptoms, these Authors directed their attention to the pre-hospital phase of the acute coronary attack and were able, with a mobile coronary-care unit, to see 294 patients within the first hour. The aim of the study was to assess the *autonomic disturbance* present during the hyperacute phase of myocardial infarction: the analysis was accomplished on 240 patients (since patients with several additional disturbances, like ventricular tachycardia, and those who were previously receiving digitalis or β-blocking agents were excluded).

Patients with sinus tachycardia and/or transient hypertension (arterial pressure 160/100 mmHg or greater) were considered to present a sympathetic overactivity. Patients with sinus bradycardia, atrioventricular block and/or transient hypotension (systolic arterial pressure 100 mmHg or less) were considered to present parasympathetic overactivity.

On the whole, 89 of the 240 patients were seen within 30 min. Only 8% of these (Webb et al. 1972) or 17% – in a subsequent evaluation (Pantridge 1978) – had normal heart rate and normal blood pressure when first seen. More than one-third showed evidence of sympathetic overactivity, while parasympathetic predominance was present in almost half of the patients. Parasympathetic overactivity occurred more frequently in association with *inferior* infarction (the term used was *posterior*). Conversely, sympathetic overactivity was more frequent in the case of *anterior* infarctions.

While this *autonomic disturbance* was present in 83% of the patients seen within 30 min, it occurred in only 56% of those seen within the second half of the first hour (Pantridge 1978).

Reflexes from the heart, of depressor (Von Bezold and Hirt 1867) or pressor (Malliani et al. 1969) nature, were considered to cause these two opposite patterns, which appeared independent of pain or pure pump failure. Remarkably, these Authors also suggested that sympathetic and parasympathetic activity could coexist, since the correction of vagal overactivity by atropine was capable of giving rise to tachycardia and transient hypertension. This finding, however, is of difficult interpretation. When atropine is administered at doses inducing peripheral muscarinic blockade, it always produces tachycardia and a simultaneous significant but slight increase in arterial pressure – in one study 7±3% (Montano et al. 1998). Hence it might be that also this finding was correctly evaluated.

The most relevant conclusion of this study, from a clinical point of view, was that both types of *autonomic disturbance* appeared to facilitate life-threatening arrhythmias.

Clinical evidence indicates that the incidence of ventricular tachycardia is higher when bradycardia accompanies myocardial infarction (Lown et al. 1967). Malignant ectopic beats may appear when the heart rate is too low. Since the incidence of bradycardia and the incidence of ventricular fibrillation are both high immediately after the onset of infarction, it has been suggested that bradycardia might be a precursor of ventricular fibrillation and an important factor in the early high mortality from acute coronary attack (Adgey et al. 1968). On the other hand, it has been often reported that hospitalized patients with sinus bradycardia have a good prognosis, suggesting a different role played by a similar low heart rate in the hyperacute and in the postacute phase. Even a few hours after the onset of the acute episode, the sinus bradycardia has been interpreted as a benign symptom (Neufeld et al. 1978).

The mechanisms according to which bradycardia and/or hypotension may have deleterious effects on atrial and ventricular function, coronary perfusion and arrhythmogenesis, are complex and still quite elusive (Pantridge et al. 1981). Conversely, it is generally accepted that an increased sympathetic activity has the possibility to increase oxygen consumption, facilitate arrhythmias (Malliani et al. 1980), and produce coronary vasoconstriction (Feigl 1983; Heusch et al. 1985; Gregorini et al. 1994).

Concerning this clinical study of paramount importance, despite its simplicity in the approach to evaluate the *autonomic disturbance,* the results of the immediate correction of autonomic alterations must also be mentioned. In fact, in addition to the early relief of pain and correction of disarrhythmias, atropine was carefully administered intravenously in cases of parasympathetic overactivity, while intravenous practolol was used to correct the sympathetic overactivity present either initially or following atropine administration. Such results appeared quite rewarding, as among the 294 patients who were seen within one hour from the onset of symptoms, mortality was less than 10%.

In view of this therapeutic success, it is truly sad that such a clinical effort was never attempted again, despite the simple principle that a physician should try to be where an acute disease is threatening a life. Cool trials have replaced this impetus to help and explore pathophysiology.

In the following years β-adrenergic receptor blocking drugs have been sporadically used in the acute phase of myocardial infarction, while their long-term administration after recovery has become highly recommended (Gottlieb et al. 1998). Similarly, in most coronary care units, atropine is currently used to treat excessive bradycardias independently of the simultaneous presence of conduction defects.

In the light of the neural circuitry outlined in Figure 7, it is hypothesized that an abnormal stimulus, like myocardial ischemia or infarction with its mechanical and chemical components, might simultaneously excite both vagal and sympathetic ventricular afferents, and hence might activate simultaneous depressor or pressor reflex mechanisms, independently of any finalistic organization of neural modulation.

Concerning the correlation between the site of the infarcted area and the type of autonomic response, a preferential distribution of vagal afferents to the inferoposterior wall of the left ventricle was postulated during experiments on dogs (Thames et al. 1978). However, several additional factors have to be evaluated, such as the proposal of a nonuniform distribution of neural afferent fibers in the ventricular myocardium, with sympathetic afferents being located mainly in the superficial epicardial layers and vagal afferents mainly in the subendocardial layers (Barber et al. 1984).

In general, these data seem to challenge the concept of an overall protective role of vagal efferent activity in the course of myocardial ischemia (Corr and Gillis 1974; De Ferrari et al. 1994).

However, in patients after myocardial infarction a large prospective study has indicated that the amplitude of the baroreflex heart rate response, which is largely effected through vagal efferents, is a favorable prognostic marker (La Rovere et al. 1998).

An experimental though acute model (Bergamaschi 1978) may synthesize the complexity of the matter. In anesthetized cats, after legation of the left anterior descending coronary artery, an electrical stimulation of the stellate ganglia (centrally disconnected) and/or the distal stump of the right vagus was performed. The simultaneous stimulation of sympathetic and parasympathetic outflows produced the most numerous and complex arrhythmias up to, in one case, ventricular fibrillation. The stimulation of the vagus alone induced bradycardia, idioventricular escape rhythm and numerous ventricular extrasystoles. In a few animals, atropine antagonized cardiac slowing and prevented the occurrence of ventricular arrhythmias, in accordance with the hypothesis by Kerzner et al (1973) that ventricular arrhythmias during vagal stimulation are rate dependent. The stimulation of the sympathetic nerves alone was the less effective arrhythmogenic intervention.

In this context, what summarized above should suffice to conclude that in pathophysiological conditions the innervated heart is likely to be in the middle of a storm which has little to do with physiological wisdom.

Transient myocardial ischemia

"A great deal has been written, but not much is as yet known, about the actual state of the cardiovascular system during attacks of angina pectoris". That was the initial sentence of a splendid article by

Sir Thomas Lewis (1931). *"Circulatory events are inconstant." "... it is usual for the pulse to remain undisturbed both in rate and in tension. On the other hand, many workers have recorded definite changes." "High rate has been found in conjunction with palpably heightened pulse tension, and less frequently with raised blood pressure readings." "Some have observed pulse slowing... ".*

Nowadays we know that angina can be accompanied by: a) hypotension and bradycardia (Guazzi et al. 1971; Robertson et al. 1985); b) hypotension and tachycardia (Guazzi et al. 1971, 1975; Maseri et al. 1978) and c) hypertension and tachycardia (Lewis 1931; Roughgarden 1966; Littler et al. 1973; Guazzi et al. 1975; Maseri et al. 1978; Robertson et al. 1985).

The usual interpretation of these different possibilities assumes that hypotension is always due to some degree of cardiac failure, that tachycardia, in such a case, reflects a baroreceptive mechanism and finally, that hypertension and tachycardia are a reflection of pain and emotion. However, these mechanisms alone would not explain those cases in which: a) hypotension is accompanied by bradycardia (Guazzi et al. 1971); b) hypertension and tachycardia occur simultaneously with electrocardiographic changes, but without pain or preceed its subjective appraisal (Littler et al. 1973; Robertson et al. 1985).

Thus, the participation of vagally mediated depressor reflexes and of sympathetically mediated excitatory reflexes appears extremely likely (Figure 7). More specifically, hypertension and tachycardia preceding or independent of pain would be the result of a reflex from the heart and not of a primary and undetermined *"vasomotor storm"* as hypothesized by Lewis (1931). It is obvious that a question of fundamental importance embraces the possibility that an increased sympathetic afferent activity can induce reflexes without pain, an issue that is analyzed subsequently in this *Chapter.*

One factor likely to influence the prevailing type of the reflex response is the extent of ischemic myocardium. This possibility was investigated (Lombardi et al. 1984) in a series of experiments carried out on anesthetized cats. In order to simplify the interaction between different reflexes, the study was performed after sino-aortic denervation. Moreover, to avoid the immediate changes in the cardiovascular regulatory mechanisms which are induced by acute baroreceptor denervation (Malliani 1980), the denervation procedure was accomplished at least one week prior to the experimental session. We produced either *global* ischemia, with transient occlusion of the left main coronary artery, or *regional* ischemia, with transient occlusion of the distal portion of the left anterior descending coronary artery. Both types of occlusion were tested before and after vagotomy.

  Global ischemia (Figure 11) before vagotomy resulted in a significant reduction of mean arterial pressure (MAP), left ventricular pressure (LVP), and left ventricular dP/dt_{max} while sympathetic efferent impulse activity was significantly augmented during the initial 15±2s of occlusion (early phase) and inhibited during the subsequent 20±2s of occlusion (late phase). Vagotomy did not modify the hemodynamic responses; however, a significant increase in sympathetic discharge was detectable during the whole occlusion period (early and late phases).

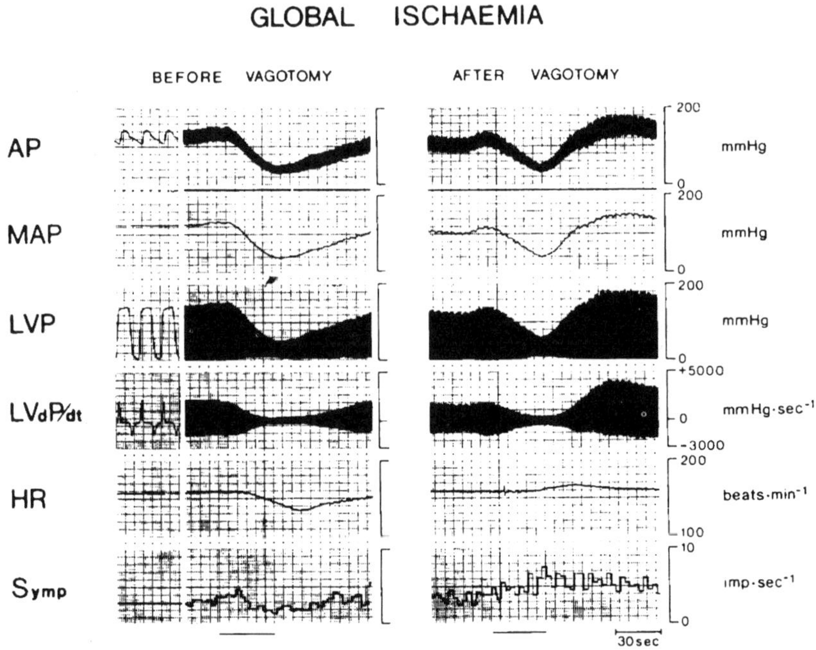

Figure 11: Effects of *global* ischemia in a cat with chronic sinoaortic denervation, before and after sectioning the vagi. The tracings represent, from top to bottom: AP, arterial pressure; MAP, mean arterial pressure; LVP, left ventricular pressure; LVdP/dt, left ventricular dP/dt; HR, heart rate; Symp, cardiac efferent sympathetic nerve activity. Bars indicate the periods of the left main coronary artery occlusions (from Lombardi et al. 1984, with permission).

Regional ischemia (Figure 12) before vagotomy resulted in a significant increase in sympathetic neural discharge and mean arterial pressure, with no changes in left ventricular function. After vagotomy the occlusion elicited a significant increase in mean arterial pressure, left ventricular pressure, left ventricular dP/dt_{max}, and efferent sympathetic neural activity. These excitatory responses were abolished after the interruption of a large part of the cardiac sympathetic afferents.

Thus, coronary artery occlusion induced hemodynamic and sympathetic reflex responses, that depended on the interaction of opposite influences mediated by the simultaneous activation of cardiac vagal and sympathetic afferents. In this experimental model the extent of *ischemic myocardium* represented a crucial factor for the prevailing type of neural response.

REGIONAL   ISCHAEMIA

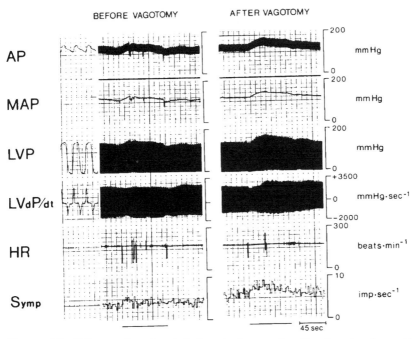

Figure 12: Effects of regional ischemia in a cat with chronic sinoaortic baroreceptor denervation, before and after sectioning the vagi. Tracings as in Figure 11. Bars indicate the periods of the left anterior descending artery occlusions (from Lombardi et al. 1984, with permission).

This would imply that transient ischemic episodes associated with hypotension and bradycardia or hypotension without the tachycardia which could be expected from a baroreceptive mechanism (i.e., events likely to reflect a vagally mediated depressor reflex), would correspond to more severe episodes of ischemia. Indeed Guazzi et al (1971) found them to be associated with acute ventricular failure. Furthermore, it is important to note that the *supernormal* phase described by Guazzi et al (1971) at the end of the ischemic episodes in humans was similar to that observed in our experiments during the recovery from *global* ischemia after vagotomy. (Figure 11).

However, pressor reflexes from the heart would be the most frequent accompaniments of less severe ischemic episodes, whether or not signaled by anginal pain (Malliani 1982, 1986). A study by Chierchia et al (1990), carried out in patients free to move and presenting frequent episodes of transient myocardial ischemia, has shown that as a rule hypertension and tachycardia seem to accompany ischemic episodes characterized by ST-segment depression, regardless of the presence or absence of pain.

It is quite clear that these neural excitatory mechanisms should not be interpreted as if they were occurring during physical exercise or an emotional experience and this is, indeed, a clear example of how physiology and pathophysiology require a different reading.

It can be concluded that experimental laboratory and clinical setting can sometimes exert a positive synergistic effect on our understanding of a complex disease.

ARTERIAL HYPERTENSION

The dawn of medical reasoning on arterial hypertension often had as a hallmark some kind of finalistic interpretation. For decades clinicians believed that elevated blood pressure forced blood through thickened arteries and arterioles, thus ensuring adequate perfusion of tissues. Consequently, they predicted that the reduction of blood pressure could only be detrimental.

As already anticipated in this Chapter, the view of essential hypertension as an abnormal *quantity* is a well-known conceptual provocation introduced by Sir George Pickering (1961) with a strong impact on contemporary pathophysiological thinking.

This new idea that essential hypertension represents a quantitative deviation from the norm, arose from the observation of the normal Gaussian frequency distribution of arterial pressure values in epidemiological surveys, while a *qualitative* disease should implicate a bimodal distribution. Obviously, this fact makes it crucial where we draw the line separating normotension from hypertension as in this way *"we can make essential hypertension as common or as rare as we wish"* (Pickering 1961).

This arbitrary choice is connected to the ancillary problem of defining, along the parallel continuum of increased mortality, another arbitrary frontier beyond which the increased quantity is considered to be significantly associated with an abnormal risk. Moreover, in view of the only partial reversibility of numerous biological phenomena, the pharmacological reduction of arterial pressure to a given level does not necessarily correspond to regaining the same risk originally associated with that given pressure. In short it should be of no surprise that a twilight zone exists, especially in view of pharmacological interventions.

Given the beauty of Pickering's idea, introducing a question without definite answer, another idea was also born during those same years of similar importance and elusiveness – that of *disease of regulation,* also known as *mosaic theory* (Page 1949). Arterial hypertension was considered to result from a constellation of facets, one or even none being more or less dominant, since more than one alteration appeared necessary to override the many mechanisms of compensatory changes.

The views of these two outstanding men were not alike at all. Page considered Pickering's idea of an *abnormal quantity* as *"primarily descriptive of a situation"* without *"particular bearing on etiology or therapy"* (Page et al. 1958). But Pickering replied (1961) that if his hypothesis had any value it was just that of being *"primarily descriptive of a situation, since this is the first phase in scientific method".*

This is to say how the absence of strong debates, as it too often happens nowadays, indicates either lack of courage or stagnancy of ideas.

Concerning the etiology of essential hypertension, Pickering considered that various factors might play an important role, including polygenic inheritance, age, environmental factors like diet and its salt content and, last but not least, factors operating through the mind.

During the normal daily life, physical activity, psychological stimuli and intense intellectual activity are as a rule associated with increases in heart rate and arterial pressure. Ingenious experiments have shown that this excitatory state can be obtained in experimental animals as well. An example deals with experiments of operating conditioning in primates – monkeys made hypertensive by a very hard operational task (Herd et al. 1969). Another intriguing experimental model was utilized by Henry et al (1975) and consisted in creating a condition of psychosocial conflict among mice confined into a net of cages and corridors that could be crossed only by one animal at a time. These environmental conditions made it possible to differentiate amongst males (socially deprived as they had been isolated during development), dominant, rival and subordinate animals. The dominant mouse was free from bites, had a glossy coat, had access to all boxes, including the female nesting cage, made frequent patrols but developed high blood pressure.

Subsequently Henry et al (1993) studied the effects of frequently repeated arousals of psychosocial competition by submitting colonies of normotensive strains of rats to continuous changes of males in group composition. The males of the most aggressive strain developed hypertension, associated with an increased heart and adrenal weight, higher values of adrenal catecholamine synthetic enzymes, myocardial fibrosis and glomerulosclerosis. Interestingly, while an enlargement of the adrenals and of the heart was present in all strains, indicating the effects of psychosocial stress, the blood pressure elevation appeared to be related to the aggressive behavior.

In the present overview the question thus becomes whether or not the mechanisms responsible for arterial pressure rise in these and similar stressful conditions bear any major similarity with the pathogenesis of essential hypertension. In simple terms, while many factors contribute to the existence of arterial pressure – including the action of the heart, the blood volume and the characteristics of the arterial tree – it is quite clear that the signal that promotes arterial pressure transient rises in physiological conditions, is of neural nature and in particular sympathetic. According to Guyton's conception (Guyton et al. 1974) *"short-term control is primarily a nervous function whereas long-term arterial blood pressure control is principally a function of the body's fluid balance system"*. This is to say that one or more factors usually contained within the background interaction undergo a progressive potentiation, according also to the *mosaic theory.*

However, given the continuum not only of the Gaussian frequency distribution, but also of the life of each individual, identifying when the pivotal role of neural mechanisms is replaced in the continuum by fluid balance leadership seems hard.

The remarkable antihypertensive efficacy of numerous and different drugs interfering at various levels with sympathetic function conversely suggests some crucial role exerted by sympathetic neural mechanisms, and not only during the early phase of the disturbance (Julius 1991). In my view it is quite tempting to conjugate Pickering's idea of an abnormal *quantity* with *quantitative and homogeneous* mechanisms acting both in physiological and pathophysiological conditions. This hypothesis would correspond to a sort of pathophysiological support to Pickering's view, expanding the concept of *continuum*. Obviously the neural mechanisms might have multifarious interactions with other factors. These might include, to take a few examples, changes in the physical properties of the vessel wall (Pickering 1961) like medial hypertrophy – the basis for the reinforcement theory proposed by Folkow (1982); insulin resistance (Ferrannini et al. 1987; Lembo et al. 1994); obesity (Landsberg 1986).

For years, however, there has been an enduring effort to demonstrate the existence of an increased sympathetic activity in human hypertension. Amongst the first probative findings, we need to recall the consistent elevation of plasma norepinephrine observed in younger hypertensives (Goldestein 1981) and the signs of an excited sympathetic discharge, detected from direct peroneal nerve recordings (Anderson et al. 1989) – recently corroborated by single unit sympathetic recordings indicating an increased discharge in early stages of hypertension (Greenwood et al. 1999). However, circulating norepinephrine represents only a small fraction of the neurotransmitter released from nerve terminals, and even the sympathetic vasoconstrictor discharge directed to the muscles does not necessarily reflect the state of sympathetic cardiac modulation. Thus, the new technique using radioisotope tracers to measure norepinephrine spillover rate has been important to detect an increased sympathetic activity to the heart and kidney in mild hypertension (Esler et al. 1990).

On clinical grounds, while interpreting an increased heart rate in the early course of hypertension might appear simple (Julius 1991), assessing the entity of sympathetic modulation of peripheral resistance has represented a truly elusive problem. Yet some traditional concepts concerning the whole organization of neural regulatory mechanisms have also represented influential barriers preventing some better understanding.

As detailed in *Chapter 1,* an increased sympathetic activity is usually attributed either to factors acting on *central command,* emotions and physical activity being the well-known paradigm, or to a decreased efficacy of *negative feedback* restraining mechanisms (Figure 1). Accordingly, quite numerous studies have attempted to obtain permanent arterial hypertension by sectioning the afferent buffering pathways supposed to exert a tonic restraining action on the centers (Cowley and Guyton 1975). It is possible that in some instances true examples of neurogenic hypertension were obtained. At the same time it appeared essential to understand how a central modulation of baroreflex mechanisms could occur (Sleight 1986) in order to explain how they could become permissive bystanders in the course of hypertension. The magic word *reset* – appropriate only for simple systems – despite the fact that the respective roles of the functional properties of supraspinal and spinal afferents and of central integration were still largely undetermined, has for decades obscured the recognition of a more complex interaction.

At any rate it appears to me at least surprising that so much effort was exclusively devoted to try to understand why neural mechanisms that should oppose hypertension were not properly acting, rather than searching, at least in parallel, for mechanisms that might simply favor the same disturbance. The first and traditional attempt was an obvious derivative of a finalist conception according to which *homeostasis* has always to prevail unless something goes really wrong, while the second view would rather accept that some mechanisms extremely purposeful in specific physiological conditions, become excessive in others – a view more simply open to what is happening and that I would define as *situational.* In terms of biological thinking, the choice is between assigning the most common disturbance of cardiovascular regulation to malfunctioning of a few thousand afferent fibers with their reflex effects, rather than to a progressive potentiation of complex patterns requiring the integration of billions of neurons.

In my view, *positive feedback* mechanisms could offer the mechanistic support to those excitatory influences largely integrated centrally and probably largely triggered by factors operating through the mind. In general, peripheral *positive feedback* reflex mechanisms might be essential to reinforce the *central command* in multifarious physiological conditions. In short they would be integrant part of that excitation which is sometimes necessary for survival, other times is the salt of life and further, especially when of unpleasant nature, generates hypertension. In terms of everyday life, Timio et al (1988) found that in 144 white nuns belonging to a secluded monastic order, followed for 20 years, arterial pressure did not increase with ageing, while it did so in control laywomen similar for all the other variables usually considered, except for their daily behavior.

However the strongest argument in favor of the likeliness of the hypothesis linking the state of excitation to peripheral *positive feedback* mechanisms, has to be found in the similarity existing between the organization of the somatic and of the autonomic nervous system (Malliani 1997). The mechanisms which produce a sustained increase in sympathetic activity may be similar to those which in the decerebrate animal are responsible for gamma-rigidity or spasticity. Sherrington (1906) found that spasticity was abolished by deafferentation. Thus it was proved that an augmented *central command* was not *per se* capable of causing a sustained increase in the postural tone, but that a peripheral spinal loop was necessary for the maintenance of the phenomenon.

To conclude with pathophysiology of arterial hypertension, while its initial phase might mainly involve the crucial drive of the mind operating through a sympathetic overactivity largely directed to the heart, the subsequent phase – sometimes concomitant with a different emotional profile – might be mainly sustained by *positive feedback* mechanisms and more directed to the peripheral vessels whose structure is progressively altered by ageing and where numerous other factors are likely to interact.

CONGESTIVE HEART FAILURE

Congestive heart failure seems to alter drastically some neural mechanisms regulating cardiovascular function. In the early investigations, where the plasma concentration of norepinephrine was taken as an index of the overall sympathetic activity, it was documented that patients with congestive heart failure had higher norepinephrine values both at rest and during exercise (Chidsey et al. 1962). Subsequently it was found that circulating levels of catecholamines were increased in heart failure in proportion to the severity of the disease (Thomas and Marks 1978) and that patients with the highest plasma concentrations had the most unfavorable prognosis (Cohn et al. 1984). With more refined techniques Eisenhofer et al (1996) observed that norepinephrine release and reuptake were both increased in the failing heart; however, the efficiency of norepinephrine reuptake was so reduced that cardiac spillover was increased disproportionately more than neuronal release of norepinephrine. At the same time the cardiac stores and the rate of vescicular leakage of norepinephrine were, respectively, 47% and 42% lower in the failing than in the normal heart. Moreover it was reported (Rundqvist et al. 1997) that in mild to moderate heart failure the cardiac adrenergic drive (assessed with norepinephrine spillover) was excited in the absence of an augmented sympathetic outflow to the kidney and skeletal muscle, which are likely to characterize more advanced stages of the disease. These last studies should exemplify, at the level of the crucial targets, the complexity of the altered sympathetic modulation.

However it has also been known for years that the reflex cardiac slowing accompanying a pressor stimulus, is greatly reduced both in man (Eckberg et al. 1971) and dogs with heart failure (Higgins et al. 1972). Furthermore, by using direct recordings of sympathetic nerve traffic Ferguson et al (1992) found that patients with moderate to severe heart failure displayed an impaired baroreflex control, not only of heart period but of muscle sympathetic nerve activity as well, and that in both cases the impairment was more pronounced during conditions of baroreceptor deactivation.

As to the mechanism leading to sympathetic excitation, for those who believe that neural cardiovascular control is exerted exclusively through *central command* and *negative feedback* mechanisms, an enigmatic ensemble of contradictory elements has to be envisaged. On the one hand, arterial hypotension, when present, appears a likely cause for an excitatory release phenomenon but, on the other hand, the congestion of thoracic low-pressure areas and the consequent activation of vagal afferents – known to play an inhibitory role (Bishop et al. 1983; Spyer 1990) – should rather oppose this sympathetic excitation. Accordingly, cumbersome explanations have been proposed for the whole process: after an initial sympathetic excitation due to the baroreceptor deactivation – secondary to the reduction in stroke volume and arterial pressure – a reduction in sensitivity of both arterial baroreceptors and cardiopulmonary vagal afferents would occur leading to their *functional denervation* and hence to their incapability of restraining the sympathetic outflow (Mancia 1990). Thus the baroreflex mechanisms would be responsible for liberating a process that would end with their suppression. Moreover, in these speculations it is hard to understand why a sympathetic reflex excitation that should have a compensatory nature – as all reflex responses promoted by a reduced restraint exerted by a *negative feedback* – should become suddenly so excessive and deleterious. At any rate, it has been recently reported (Ando et al. 1997) that patients with heart failure and *pulsus alternans* presented also a correlated alternation in the discharge of the muscle sympathetic nerve activity, clearly indicating the existence of brisk baroreflex mechanisms.

However, some clinical knowledge and well proved experimental findings may offer a different and more sound interpretation of the mechanisms leading to sympathetic excitation also in the presence of an active baroreflex system.

Beginning with clinical notions, every physician knows or should know that acute heart failure accompanied by pulmonary congestion is quite often characterized by an increase in both arterial pressure and heart rate: the patient in addition is sweating and , on the whole, is one of the most dramatic examples of sympathetic overactivity. Dyspnea may easily explain the emotional arousal and hence the sympathetic excitation: however, the observation of tachycardia and hypertension preceding the dyspnea is common, making unlikely the initial role of both baroreflex deactivation and central emotional excitation.

On the basis of the experimental evidence summarized in *Chapter 1*, we have advanced for several years an alternative hypothesis (Malliani and Pagani 1983): the increase in cardiac dimensions and filling pressures and the congestion of the low-pressure thoracic vascular areas would activate cardiovascular sympathetic afferents, which are extremely sensitive to such changes (Lombardi et al. 1976; Malliani 1982), and hence elicit a state of early sympathetic reflex excitation. Figures 7-9 in *Chapter 1* exemplify the neural circuits and some of the experimental evidence supporting this hypothesis. According to it, the progressive sympathetic excitation during the evolution of the disease would be mediated by *both* activation of cardiopulmonary sympathetic afferents and arterial baroreceptor deactivation and this would explain the marked degree of such sympathetic overactivity.

Some aspects of these abnormal responses can be detected also in the course of human pathophysiological investigation. As an example, a paradoxical increase in forearm vascular resistance has been observed in patients with mild heart failure during saline load (Volpe et al. 1991), suggesting that the reflex excitatory response was due to the stimulation of cardiovascular low-pressure receptors rather than to the deactivation of some *negative feedback* reflexogenic area.

The finding that the activation of afferent sympathetic fibers is not only capable of exciting the sympathetic outflow but also of blunting the baroreflex bradycardia in both acute (Gnecchi Ruscone et al. 1987) and chronic experiments (Pagani et al. 1982) represents a further crucial link between *negative* and *positive feedback* mechanisms. This corresponds, in conceptual terms, to another overturning of the traditional view: the sympathetic excitation would be the cause of blunted baroreflex mechanisms and not only the consequence of their deactivation or reduced sensitivity. This new perspective is also supported by the experiments of Zucker's group (Brändle et al. 1996; Wang and Zucker 1996; Ma et al. 1997) on dogs with congestive heart failure, indicating that the afferent sympathetic excitation and its central regulation might have a crucial role in mediating the initial sympathetic overactivity.

In conclusion, also in the case of heart failure the excitation of cardiovascular sympathetic afferents would play a pivotal role in leading to an abnormal excitatory state independent of any *homeostatic* design.

CARDIAC PAIN

"There is perhaps no symptom familiar to clinicians that has given rise to more speculation than that of anginal pain". Lewis (1932a), the author of this sentence, was merited with having initiated a critical evaluation of the link between muscular ischemia and pain but, as it often occurs, better knowledge was soon transformed into a choral certainty. Entire generations of physicians lived, and still perhaps do, with the conviction that acute myocardial ischemia, as a rule, leads to pain. Cardiac pain hence became a reliable warning symptom, reflecting tissue damage and its natural history.

In general, the reasons for attributing to pain a protective value to the organism were based on common sense well before the existence of specific nociceptors was claimed: and although to the body noxious does not necessarily mean pain and pain does not necessarily mean damage, the common experience remains that it is rare to heavily injure a part of the body without pain. If this is so on the soma, it surely does not apply to the viscous and, in particular, to the heart (Malliani et al. 1989).

This part of the *Chapter* will deal with the argumentation that a well conceived alarm system from the heart does not exist, and this will be a further indication that pathophysiology does not reflect a finalistic design.

The symptom and the traditional interpretation

It is a symptom of antique description. The philosopher Lucius Annaeus Seneca, who suffered from chest pain likely to have been anginal, perhaps slightly related to the not totally rewarding task of being Nero's teacher, wrote about twenty centuries ago: *"The attack is short and the impetus like a storm; it usually ceases within an hour: who could indeed be expiring for a long time? I have experienced all other illnesses and dangers ... to have any malady is only to be sick, to have this is to be dying. Therefore doctors call it 'meditation of death'"* (Epistulae morales ad Lucilium, Liber VI, Epistula II).

The afferent pathway

The notion that the afferent fibers running in the cardiac sympathetic nerves were the only essential pathway for the transmission of cardiac pain arose from observations on both humans and experimental animals.

In man thoracic sympathectomy or section of the higher thoracic dorsal roots was found to be a maneuver capable of relieving anginal pain (Jonnesco 1921; White 1957), while stellate ganglionectomy could abolish behavioral reactions accompanying coronary occlusion in acute experiments (Sutton and Lueth 1930). Observations which were consistent with Langley's statement (1903) that *"most of the afferent fibres, which on electrical stimulation give rise to pain, pass by the sympathetic strands and not by the vagus"*. From the heart these afferent nerve fibers run to the spinal cord through the cardiac nerves, the upper five thoracic sympathetic ganglia, the white rami communicantes or, to a minor extent, the grey rami and, lastly, the upper five thoracic dorsal roots (White 1957).

In the spinal cord some impulses mediated by the sympathetic afferent pathway seem to converge together with impulses from somatic thoracic structures onto the same ascending spinal neurons. In this way, the original *"convergence-projection theory"* proposed by Ruch (1955) and supported by the experiments by Foreman and Ohata (1980) provides the most likely explanation for cardiac referred pain. In addition, some contribution by vagal afferent fibers in the mediation of cardiac nociception cannot be dismissed too hastily. Indeed, the anginal pain referred to the jaw, head and neck, more frequent after sympathectomy – the phenomenon of *migration of pain* (Lindgren and Olivecrona 1947), – may indicate an additional central site, besides the spinal cord, where the mechanisms for referred pain may be activated, in this case by cardiac vagal afferent fibers. Moreover, even when nociception would be transmitted through afferent sympathetic fibers, an important modulatory role might be exerted by vagal afferents (Ammons et al. 1983).

The adequate stimulus

One day William Harvey and Charles I, a highly sophisticated team, touched the beating heart of the young Viscount Montgomery, incredibly exposed through a large thoracic wound, and they had to acknowledge *"that the heart was without the sense of touch; for the youth never knew when we touched his heart except for the sight or the sensation he had through the external integument"* (Willis 1847). This experiment, often cited for its fallacy, provided the dawn of a future certitude: touch and pain were not to be equated.

However, it was not until around the time of the French Revolution that cardiac pain was indisputably described and attributed to coronary disease by a group of cooperating investigators, namely Heberden, Jenner, and Parry, as well as John Hunter who suffered from angina. In Heberden's view coronary disease was of spasmodic nature and Jenner believed that spasms were painful (Rinzler 1952). Even more astonishing was Parry's theory that *"rigidity of the coronary arteries"* could produce a temporal interference with the blood supply required by the vigorous action of the heart, thus causing *"syncope"*, preceded by a notable anxiety or pain in the region of the heart. In short, a reduction of coronary blood flow was linked with weakness of the heart or with pain from the heart.

Within the first hypothesis that a reduced blood supply could cause weakness of action, we have to appreciate the contribution by

Burns who, well acquainted with Parry's ideas, wrote in 1809 that *"a limb round which we have with a moderate degree of tightness applied a ligature can only support its action for a very short time; consequently fails and sinks into a state of quiescence. A heart, the coronary vessels of which are cartilaginous or ossified, is in nearly a similar condition",* as quoted by Lewis (1932a) who also pointed out that Potain was really the first, in 1866, to clearly compare the pain arising from the heart and from an ischemic muscle. Subsequently the second proposition appeared to progressively consolidate: cardiac pain and not cardiac weakness was the crucial marker of a reduction of coronary blood flow.

When Sherrington (1906) individuated in the *"nocuous"* event, threatening the integrity of a tissue, the stimulus capable, by definition, of triggering nociception, he furnished more of a general concept for the interpretation of somatic pain than a universal key for predicting all types of nociception. For instance, as to the heart, in the same period it became known that *"in acute endocarditis pain is rarely present, and ulceration of valves or of the wall may proceed to a most extreme degree without any sensory disturbance"* (Osler 1910). That is to say that for the heart an ambiguous relationship between damage and pain has long been known.

Around the thirties the problem of the adequate stimulus for cardiac pain was sharply focused in experimental terms. On the side of chemical stimuli the foreground was occupied by Lewis' (1932a) appealing proposal of a *"factor P"*, capable of inducing nociception and accumulating in the tissue spaces when a muscle is exercising under ischemic conditions.

On the mechanical side Colbeck (1903) had had a stimulating intuition: *"the hypothesis I suggest ascribes the pain experienced in the anginal paroxism to localised distension and stretching of the ventricular wall"*. Subsequently, Tennant and Wiggers (1935) suggested the stretch undergone during systole by the ventricular regions acutely deprived of blood supply as the abnormal mechanical stimulus. At about the same time, Martin and Gorham (1938) showed that an appropriate mechanical stretch of the coronary arteries could produce *"pseudoaffective reactions"* in animals in absence of myocardial ischemia. It is still worthwhile to reconsider their words: *"Our experiments do not offer any direct evidence to disprove the possibility of the generally accepted theory that ischemia is the cause of cardiac pain, but they do prove that pain may be produced mechanically in the absence of any chemical stimulus".*

Although the problem was far from being solved, Lewis' prestige transformed his hypothesis into a common belief and the abnormal accumulation of chemical substances became the nub of the traditional view of how the adequate stimulus is engendered in the ischemic myocardium.

"Intensity" or "specificity"

We are here merely by two old hypotheses which, however, have often been adopted as doctrines (Figure 13).

The *'intensity'* mechanism, the most obvious and probably the first to be formulated, assumes that pain is caused by an excessive stimulation of receptive structures (Gooddy 1957). In the dawn of modern biology, Erasmus Darwin (1794) somehow equated pain with excessive sensation: *"In these cases the violent contractions of fiber produce pain. . . and this pain constitutes an additional kind or quantity of excitement"* (Section XII: 4).

Alternatively, pain may be considered a *'specific'* sensation (Perl 1971): that is, the product of the excitation of a well defined nociceptive apparatus, the functional characteristics of which make it responsive only to a limited class of events, *'nocuous'* (Sherrington 1906) stimuli, that threaten the integrity of a tissue. The predecessor of this view is probably to be found in the doctrine of specific energies by Johannes Müller (1840): he advanced the idea that different types of nerve fibers respond to different stimuli because of their special receptive structures; as a consequence, the activity in each particular nerve fiber always gives rise to the same sensation, whether the stimulus acts externally or internally.

After these premises, it should be clear that the *"specificity"* theory was also in the epicenter of the traditional interpretation of cardiac pain. Indeed, the assignment of the afferent sympathetic path to the exclusive transmission of pain coincided with the most committed conceptualization of a specific nociceptive channel, not only in the usual terms of a peculiar contingent of small diameter afferent fibers (Perl 1971) but as the whole sensory input contained in an ensemble of nerves. Hence, the sympathetic sensory endings within the heart were equated to *"specific"* nociceptors.

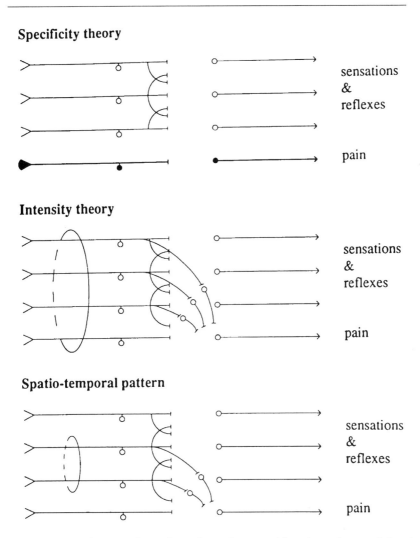

Specificity theory

Intensity theory

Spatio-temporal pattern

Figure 13: Schema of various hypotheses addressing the peripheral transmission of the algogenic code. According to *specificity theory* (upper diagram) specific nociceptors (black filled neuron) are connected with a central pathway specifically assigned to the transmission of painful sensations. According to *intensity theory* (middle diagram), pain arises from an excessive stimulation of peripheral neurons normally subserving the transmission of other sensory modalities. According to the *spatio/temporal pattern* hypothesis, pain would arise when an intense peripheral stimulation is concentrated and not homogeneously distributed thus activating the central pattern transmitting nociception. In these two last hypotheses a central pathway specific for pain transmission is not required. (Modified from Handwerker 1984).

The new experimental findings
Do cardiac specific nociceptors exist?

This question can be explored experimentally. Peripheral sensors, purely nociceptive in function, should have no or very erratic background discharge (Perl 1971) as a consequence of their high threshold, which renders them unresponsive to normal events and excitable only with strong stimuli likely to be noxious. Thus the *recruitment* of their silent fibers by a peripheral stimulus could represent an unambiguous signal to the centers. It is well known, for instance, that on the somatic side there is a population of afferent fibers innervating the skin, which have receptors that seem to fit the criteria for specific nociceptors (Perl 1971): no background discharge and recruitment only with strong mechanical or thermal stimuli.

In this context an intense electrophysiologic investigation, as described in *Chapter 1*, was carried out into the properties of either the small myelinated or unmyelinated ventricular sympathetic afferent fibers, i.e., the afferent fibers that are more likely to convey cardiac nociception. It was found that these fibers possess a mechanosensitivity that makes them tonically active and responsive to normal hemodynamic events. Coronary occlusion or intracoronary administration of bradykinin, i.e., possible algesic stimuli, increased markedly their tonic impulse activity, but a recruitment of silent afferent fibers could not be appreciated (Figure 3).

Adenosine as well markedly excited their impulse activity and potentiated their responsiveness to coronary occlusion, but was incapable of recruiting silent afferent sympathetic fibers (Gnecchi Ruscone et al. 1995). Accordingly, the conceptual frame of the problem seems unaltered by replacing bradykinin with adenosine, in order to claim the existence of specific cardiac nociceptors (Sylvén et al. 1986; Crea et al. 1990).

It is concluded that the *"intensity"* mechanism appears as the most likely candidate to account for the properties of the neural substrate subserving cardiac nociception (Malliani 1982, 1986; Malliani and Lombardi 1982; Malliani et al. 1989). Hence, ventricular sympathetic sensory endings are not *specific* nociceptors, but *low-threshold polymodal receptors*.

Experimental preparations and adequacy of the stimulus

Pain is a conscious experience that can be explored only indirectly with experimental preparations; therefore, different opinions on peripheral nociceptive mechanisms are often the result of different preparations.

In animals recovering from anesthesia or in decerebrate acute preparations, it is quite easy to obtain *"pseudoaffective reflexes"* (Woodworth and Sherrington 1904) by applying noxious stimuli to the heart. Thus, Sutton and Lueth (1930) observed that traction on a ligature placed around a coronary artery could elicit *"evidence of severe pain"*.

Leaving unsolved whether the possible adequate stimulus for cardiac pain is mainly mechanical (Martin and Gorham 1938), chemical (Lewis 1932a; Baker et al. 1980) or a mixture of both, I shall rather focus on the fundamental fact whether a similar stimulus appears algogenic or not, depending only on the specific experimental set.

The nonapeptide bradykinin was likely to furnish a remarkable tool for the experimental analysis of this subject, as it was considered the most powerful of natural algogenic substances, and able to be quantified when used as a stimulus (Lombardi et al. 1981).

Indeed, the initial observations by Guzman et al (1962) appeared extremely sound and easy to interpret when they reported that intracoronary injections of bradykinin produced overt pain reactions very effectively in dogs recovering from recent surgery.

As already reported in *Chapter I,* we have analyzed the reflex hemodynamic effects of the chemical stimulation with bradykinin of the cardiac sensory innervation in conscious dogs after full recovery from the operation necessary for instrumentation (Pagani et al. 1985b).

In these animals the injections of graded doses of bradykinin in either the left anterior descending or the circumflex coronary artery consistently produced gradual increases in systemic arterial pressure and heart rate as well as left ventricle pressure and dP/dt (Figure 14, right panel).

It is important to point out that these changes were never accompanied by any pain reaction, as expressed by agitation and vocalization of the animals. In this study the amounts of bradykinin injected into the cannulated coronary artery ranged from 10 ng/kg (the threshold dose for the response) to 3 µg/kg. When this latter very large dose was used, however, the direct vasodilatory effects of the drug prevailed and hypotension and tachycardia were observed, again in absence of any pain reaction. A similar pressor response, in the absence of pain reaction, was also seen when bradykinin was injected into the pericardial sac (Pagani et al. 1985b).

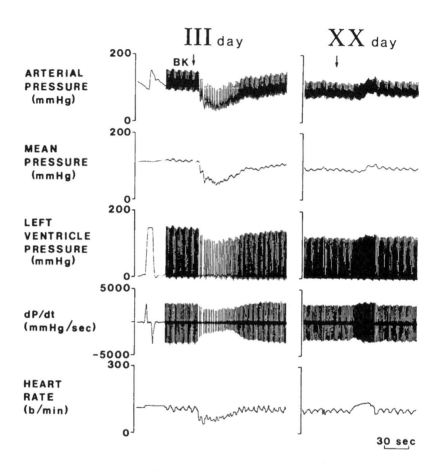

Figure 14: Contrasting effects of intracoronary bradykinin (100 ng/kg) in a conscious dog when examined early (left panel) and late (right panel) after surgery. Note that while a depressor response was obtained on the third post-operative day, it reverted to a pressor response at a time of complete recovery from surgery (20th post-operative day). (From Malliani et al. 1986a, with permission).

The importance of recovery from anesthesia and recent surgery in explaining the apparent discrepancy with the finding by Guzman et al (1962), was demonstrated by experiments performed soon after surgery, when recovery of the animals was still incomplete. Injections of bradykinin into the coronary bed of nine animals during the first week after surgery provoked either an early depressor (Figure 14, left panel) or a pressor response, which became the usual constant pressor response at a time of complete recovery from surgery (Figure 14, right panel). Moreover, three of the nine dogs exhibited vocalization and agitation suggesting a pain reaction, in response to the bradykinin injections performed during the first week after surgery – and this occurrence is illustrated in Figure 14. Such a reaction was no longer present when the animals were tested later on, after complete recovery from surgery (Pagani et al. 1985b).

Absence of pain was also reported (Barron and Bishop 1982) in relation to intracoronary injections of veratridine, a non-physiological compound likely to stimulate directly (Paintal 1971) the nerve fibers, and surely capable of activating both vagal (Von Bezold and Hirt 1867), and sympathetic afferent fibers (Uchida and Murao 1974c; Nishi et al. 1977; Baker et al. 1980; Lombardi et al. 1981).

The observation that under appropriate experimental conditions an excitation of the cardiac sensory supply – likely to be massive did not elicit pain, appears as a total defeat for the *"specificity"* theory, at least if nociceptors were postulated to be exquisitely sensitive to bradykinin (Baker et al. 1980). On the other hand, the *"intensity"* theory as well does not explain in simple terms the lack of induction of pain.

The new hypothesis

As a working hypothesis we propose a modified version of the intensity mechanism. Cardiac pain would result from the extreme excitation of a spatially restricted population of sympathetic afferents (Malliani 1982, 1986; Malliani et al. 1989) (Figure 13). The result shown in Figure 15 could be interpreted in this sense: indeed, a peculiar position maintained in this experiment by the coronary cannula, lying just outside the wall of the vessel and below the adventitia, determined that each minute injection distended a limited portion of the adventitia. It should be noted that a similarly marked pressor, inotropic and heart rate response was observed with injections of either bradykinin or saline. The animal displayed overt pain reactions to every trial, independently of the pressor effect, as they persisted when the hypertensive responses were blunted by α-adrenergic receptor blockade with phentolamine (Figure 15, panels B and C). The pain reaction being similarly induced by both bradykinin and saline, the effective stimulus was likely to be the mechanical distension of the adventitia.

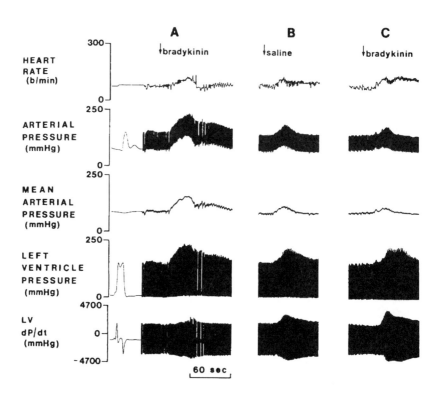

Figure 15: Effects of mechanical distension of the adventitia of the left circumflex coronary artery produced in a conscious dog by sub-adventitial injections of either bradykinin or saline. Similar pain reactions (vocalization and agitation) were observed even though the pressor response was blunted by α-adrenergic receptor blockade with phentolamine (1 mg/kg between A and B; again between B and C). LV, left ventricle. (From Malliani et al. 1986a)

One experiment should not be the basis for a theory, but it is well known that experimental causality has often offered new perspectives on a problem. The implications of this hypothesis could be relevant. A spatially restricted mechanical abnormality localized in the myocardium or in the abundantly innervated coronary arteries could lead to pain more efficiently than a more widely distributed myocardial ischemia with its chemical components. Thus, coronary spasm could be a highly effective stimulus, or some local muscular dyssynergy. Obviously, I am not equating anginal pain, for which mechanical factors could be prevalent, and pain in the course of myocardial infarction, when the interaction between accumulation of chemical and mechanical factors is likely to reach its maximum.

According to this hypothesis, when the activation of the cardiac sympathetic afferent fibers is widely and homogeneously distributed, as in the case of intracoronary injections of bradykinin or, more currently, during a marked increase in arterial pressure, central inhibitory modulations (Wall and Melzack 1989) will prevent the onset of pain. Conversely, by inducing a localized somatic afferent barrage, recent thoracic surgery could decisively contribute – through mechanisms of convergence at spinal level – to the genesis of the peculiar algogenic code.

Pathophysiological observations

It has been well documented that in patients exhibiting spontaneous and reversible ECG changes typical of episodes of transient myocardial ischemia, the hemodynamic profile of the crises can appear substantially similar whether or not they are accompanied by pain (Guazzi et al. 1971, 1975; Maseri et al. 1978; Chierchia et al 1990). Careful analysis revealed that several factors are likely to be implicated in the genesis of pain, such as duration of the episode or severity of ischemia. For instance, ischemic crises were usually painless when shorter than 3 minutes and associated with increases in left ventricular filling pressure less than 7 mm Hg (Maseri et al. 1985). However, above these values the onset of pain was unpredictable. In brief, duration and severity of ischemia appeared necessary but not sufficient in themselves. Be that as it may, the temporal sequence of ischemic episodes – sometimes more than one per hour, about 70 percent of which unaccompanied by pain – seems to furnish a most intriguing clinical puzzle.

Similarly, in conscious chronically instrumented dogs Rimoldi et al (1990) noticed that coronary occlusion elicited signs of pain in 5 out of 11 animals, but always after 2 min occlusion (unpublished observations).

The elusive link

The link between pain and tissue damage is the basis of a conception that assigns to pain a primordial and protective value for living organisms. While this principle seems corroborated by most common observations on somatic injuries, it seems unlikely to be valid, as such, for the heart where the link is much more elusive.

This elusiveness has been attributed to a *"defective anginal warning system"* (Cohn 1980). In my opinion warning is a state of consciousness that depends not only on afferent inputs but also on the degree of awareness and culture: similarly cardiac pain embraces a whole spectrum of sensations (Procacci and Zoppi 1989). In this regard, it is worthwhile recalling an old debate between James Mackenzie, who claimed that surgical relief of cardiac pain would endanger patient's life because angina was an important warning symptom of overexertion, and White (1957) who maintained that even after cardiac sympathectomy the patient continues to experience warning signals such as constriction, dyspnea (Seneca's "difficult breath," *suspirium),* and palpitation. In short, warning is unlikely to depend on a unique afferent pathway when the warning signal does not belong to a specific sense. It may at this stage be worth quoting a sentence by Reid and De Witt Andrus (1925) I consider truly remarkable for its anticipating wisdom: *"Nobody believes that all pain originating in and around the heart is always due to the same cause"'*.

In *Chapter 1* it has been amply reported that cardiovascular sympathetic afferent fibers are tonically active and mediate reflexes that are mainly excitatory in nature, with *positive feedback* characteristics. It is thus likely that the primary role of this afferent channel is to contribute to the neural regulation of circulatory functions. The capability of their cardiac sensory terminals to detect ischemic damage or abnormal changes related to it, and their connections with the central structures elaborating the perception of pain has, on pathophysiologic finalistic grounds and in the absence of better knowledge, suggested as basic an accessory function. However, again by the Darwinian or a similar hypothesis, it is hard to understand the biologic strategy and hence the development of a system providing the wild animal with hundreds of fibers, exclusively designed for signaling unlikely coronary emergencies. Even more surprising is a warning system that lets so many dangers filter: this porosity seems to denote a different biological purpose. More simply, physiology and pathophysiology are unlikely to share the same finalistic organization.

CONCLUSIONS

I think that pain, apart from its psychical adjunct, can be considered as a multifactorial entity (Malliani et al. 1989). To simplify, three different levels of interactions can be described.

1. At the level of the peripheral stimulus, the effective nociceptive code remains a mystery. As a working hypothesis we proposed (Malliani 1986; Malliani et al. 1989) a modified version of the intensity mechanism (Figure 13). Cardiac pain would result from the extreme excitation of a spatially restricted population of afferent sympathetic fibers: hence, it would stem from an afferent code based upon a peculiar *spatio/temporal pattern*. More explicitly, an intense excitation of afferent sympathetic fibers would be more likely to reach the effectiveness of a nociceptive code when characterized by spatial heterogeneity. Thus, besides the extension and severity of ischemia, which would determine the background of afferent excitation, further crucial stimulation of the sensory endings could occur in those regions where mechanical stretching is maximal, or where chemical compounds accumulate to further excite the sensory endings, or where an abnormal vasomotion takes place; all these events could contribute importantly to the spatial heterogeneity.

2. At the level of the spinal cord, neural mechanisms are capable of either accentuating (Foreman and Ohata 1980) or reducing nociception. The latter mechanisms would comprise those activated by transcutaneous electrical nerve stimulation (Mannheimer et al. 1986) or dorsal column stimulation (Murphy and Giles 1987). Cardiac vagal afferents, which might have an inhibitory effect on spinal transmission (Foreman 1986), are likely to be co-activated during the same normal or abnormal cardiac events that excite sympathetic afferents (Bishop et al. 1983). Finally, endogenous peptides are also located at this level (Weidinger et al. 1986). The challenge with this new legion of candidates is discriminating between artificial possibilities and pathophysiological mechanisms likely to occur.

Some attempts in pain research (Wall 1985) should be centered on these two levels: the peripheral input and the spinal cord integration. As no spinal pathway has been found to carry exclusively visceral sensation, but rather convergent information from the soma and from the viscera, it is likely that the processing of either input could exert a reciprocal influence on the other.

3. The central level, at very least, governs cognition, attention, situational context, and psychological distress (Barsky 1986). This complexity level should be considered when evaluating some interesting findings, such as the facilitatory role of tachyarrhythmias on the occurrence of pain during ischemic episodes (Biagini et al. 1988), because the arrhythmias could represent an additional mechanical stimulus or, alternatively, a further element of psychological distress. On similar grounds, the subjective threshold for pain (Procacci et al. 1976; Droste et al. 1986) could depend upon various mechanisms. However, while individual variations in this threshold might provide some explanation for asymptomatic patients, it gives no clue to the most frequently occurring events in anginal patients, namely the asymptomatic episodes versus the symptomatic ones.

In this context it can be accepted that in clinics, cardiac pain sometimes appearing as an ally, is more often just an unreliable witness of some damage. In terms of our *spatio/temporal pattern* hypothesis no stimulus acting on the heart should be expected, because of its quality, to elicit pain as a rule.

Physiologists know that sensation is an abstraction, not a replication of the real world. Clinicians should be aware that cardiac pain more than an abstraction is only a possibility, and yet a cornerstone symptom.

PHARMACOLOGICAL CONSIDERATIONS

In the early sixties, Sir James W. Black developed propranolol, thus realizing a major breakthrough in the design of a receptor antagonist. The drug, expected to reduce heart's demand for oxygen, was initially used in the treatment of exertional angina. By now β-blockers are considered to be one of the first choices in the treatment of arterial hypertension, while gaining an increasing consensus in the therapy for heart failure (Packer 1998). Last but not least, considerable evidence indicates remarkable effects of β-blockers long-term administration to patients after myocardial infarction (Gottlieb et al. 1998). The mechanisms of this wide therapeutic efficacy are still quite elusive, although it seems obvious to suppose some blunting effect exerted on sympathetic modulation, likely to be deleteriously increased. Conversely, it is unlikely that the underlying sympathetic overactivity in these different conditions may subserve a compensatory function as in such a case its attenuation would be harmful. This is the reason for briefly alluding, in this context, to the hypothesis linking neural mechanisms and therapeutic efficacy of β-blockers.

Mechanisms of action of β-blockers

The mechanisms usually considered are centered on the efferent side of sympathetic modulation (Packer 1998). However Uchida and Murao (1974d) reported that propranolol reduces the activation of left ventricular sympathetic afferent fibers during experimental coronary artery occlusion. Subsequently Thorén (1977) observed that propranolol markedly attenuates the increase in discharge of left ventricular receptors with nonmyelinated vagal afferents during rises in left ventricular end-diastolic pressure induced by graded aortic constriction. This effect was attributed to the reduction in ventricular contractility induced by the drug. Thames confirmed (1980) this observation and further pointed out that the influence of changes in contractility and systolic pressure becomes evident mainly when end-diastolic pressure is raised.

An additional evidence that a β-adrenergic receptor blocking drug can reduce the neural afferent input from the cardiovascular system to the neural centers, was obtained by Lombardi and co-workers (1986). In these experiments we recorded the impulse activity from afferent sympathetic fibers with aortic and pulmonary vein sensory endings, i.e. from high- and low-pressure vascular receptors, during aortic constrictions leading to an increase in both aortic and left atrial pressure. The responsiveness of these afferents to similar increases in pressure was drastically decreased after β-blockade administration: however, it could not be determined whether this reduced responsiveness was due to an alteration of the fine characteristics of the hemodynamic stimulus or to a direct effect of the drug on the vessels elasticity, as it is known that changes in the mechanical function of the vessel wall can affect the transducer properties of the nerve endings (Brown 1980).

On the whole, considering the *positive feedback* characteristics of the sympatho-sympathetic reflexes, β-blockers have the possibility of blunting sympathetic modulation by acting on both the input and output of the circuit.

A hypothesis on β-blockade therapeutic efficacy

The progressive attenuation of *positive feedback* reflex mechanisms may explain the truly puzzling observation that β-blockers are capable of decreasing systemic vascular resistance (Packer 1998). This change in this hemodynamic variable should play a role of paramount importance in the therapy of both essential hypertension and heart failure.

On the other hand, in patients after myocardial infarction the attenuation of sympathetic excitatory reflexes during eventual ischemic episodes may be the cause for the reduction of life-threatening arrhythmias and reinfarctions. In addition, premature ventricular contractions are associated to marked increases in sympathetic discharge largely related to baroreceptive mechanisms (Lombardi et al. 1989). Thus numerous possibilities exist of creating vicious or virtuous circles between arrhythmias and sympathetic excitation. However, despite the favorable indications provided by quite large studies (Gottlieb et al. 1998), the theoretical possibility remains that in some cases β-blockade might worsen a life-threatening bradyarrhythmia (Malliani et al. 1980) in the course of an acute coronary event. On the other hand, the effects of dumping an excessive sympathetic drive might be of benefit also in the presence of a vagal overactivity. And finally there is also the paradoxical possibility that simultaneously depressor reflexes might be blunted by the action of the drug on their afferent limb, mostly represented by vagal afferents.

Needless to say that we have no information yet on all these possible interactions that appear indeed of vital importance, in the true sense of the word.

As one can see the finalistic design has faded out. In pathophysiology, quite often, one would say: *"it happened to be the case"*.

Chapter 3
THE SYMPATHOVAGAL BALANCE EXPLORED IN THE FREQUENCY DOMAIN

The neural regulation of circulatory function is mainly effected through the interplay of the sympathetic and vagal outflows, which are tonically and phasically modulated by means of the interaction of at least three major factors: *central command* (or *central integration*), peripheral inhibitory reflex mechanisms (with *negative feedback* characteristics), and peripheral excitatory reflex mechanisms (with *positive feedback* characteristics) (Figure 1).

To study this whole interplay only through the action of single reflexes appears an unsound illusion, since the fragmented pieces of knowledge are difficult if not impossible to reassemble into a unitary conception. Simplified but general hypotheses might be necessary. In this respect the sympathovagal interaction might furnish an appealing conceptual model.

The sympathovagal balance

In most physiological conditions, the activation of either sympathetic or vagal outflow is accompanied by the inhibition of the other (hence the concept of *balance*, as a horizontal beam pivoted at its center) (Malliani 1999a; Malliani et al. 1991a, 1998). This is true for reflexes arising not only predominantly from the arterial baroreceptive areas but also from the heart. For instance, we have already seen in *Chapter 1* that the stimulation of cardiac sympathetic afferents induces reflex sympathetic excitation and vagal inhibition, whereas the opposite effect is elicited by stimulating cardiac vagal afferents (Schwartz et al. 1973). This reciprocal reflex organization, alluding to a synergistic design, seems instrumental to the fact that sympathetic excitation and simultaneous vagal inhibition, or viceversa, are both presumed to contribute to the increase or decrease of cardiac performance to implement various behaviors.

The schema of Figure 1 has thus been slightly modified into a version (Figure 16) in which the central and peripheral mechanisms do not regulate a single autonomic outflow but rather a complex interaction exemplified by *sympathovagal balance*.

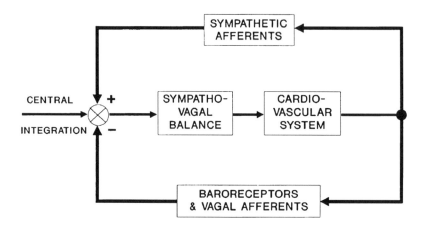

Figure 16: Schema of opposing feedback mechanisms that, in addition to central integration, regulate the state of sympathovagal balance. See text and Appendix. (From Malliani et al. 1991a, with permission).

It is the purpose of this *Chapter* to demonstrate that this interaction can be broadly explored by assessing cardiovascular rhythmicity with an appropriate methodology. In fact, variable phenomena such as heart period and arterial blood pressure can be described not only as a function of time (i.e. in the *time domain*), but also as the sum of elementary oscillatory components, defined by their frequency and amplitude (i.e. in the *frequency domain*).

Neural and cardiovascular rhythms as markers of functional states

Rhythmicity is an intrinsic property of the nervous system. Various rhythms can be markers of normal events, such as wakefulness or sleep, and of abnormal conditions, such as epilepsy. However, a rhythm is rarely unequivocally linked with a function: thus an atropinized cat can walk around with an electroencephalogram simulating placid sleep. On the other hand, circulation and respiration, strictly related transport functions, are both based on discontinuous events and oscillations of various orders characterize them, in particular cardiovascular variables. It has been a traditional endeavor of experimental physiology to describe such oscillations, to investigate their causes and, more recently, the links existing between neural and cardiovascular rhythms, in view of a possible functional significance. Surely the oldest are the observations on rhythmic fluctuations of systemic arterial pressure, as they started with Reverend Stephen Hales' (1733) experiment during which oscillations of first and second order were observed, i.e., those related to cardiac cycle and respiration (Figure 17).

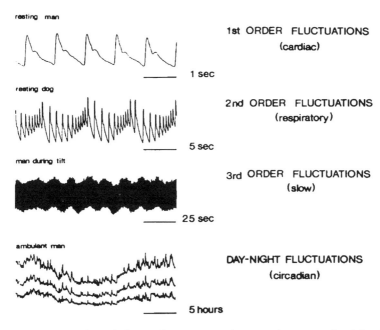

Figure 17: Examples of the various waves that can be recognized in the arterial pressure tracing. Notice the decrease of time scale in the progression of fluctuation order. The arterial pressure in ambulant man was recorded with a high-fidelity technique (Pagani et al. 1986a): in this case the tracings represent from top to bottom the systolic, the mean and the diastolic pressure values.

As to the third-order oscillations, i.e. those with a period apparently longer than the respiratory cycle, Koepchen (1984) has reviewed their history and the various interpretations that have flourished around them: according to his conclusions we shall assume the waves described by Sigmund Mayer (1876) with a period of about 10 seconds as the prototype of the third-order oscillations of arterial pressure. However, the period of this type of oscillation is highly variable.

With regard to the rhythms discernible in the discharge of the autonomic outflow, Adrian and coworkers (1932) were the first to record from sympathetic nerves an efferent impulse activity displaying a rhythm in phase with cardiac cycle and respiration. Several decades had to elapse before Fernandez de Molina and Perl (1965) observed, in spinal cats, rhythmic increases in sympathetic discharge simultaneous to slow arterial pressure waves.

As to the impulse activity of vagal efferent fibers, the existence of cardiac and respiratory rhythms was also reported (Jewett 1964; Kunze 1975) before the description of an additional rhythm in phase with third order arterial pressure oscillations (Kollai and Koizumi 1981).

There has been much debate, during the years, on the origin of these neural rhythms along two fundamental hypotheses. Indeed, they could depend on either an afferent peripheral modulation or autochthonous oscillating properties of the central nervous system. In order to give an example of a pioneering point of view, Adrian et al. (1932) concluded, on sympathetic rhythms, that *"it seems most likely that the (cardiac) grouping must be dependent on the rhythmic sensory outbursts reaching the brain stem"*, while the *"respiratory grouping is due to a direct action of the respiratory centre on the vasomotor centre, for it persists in the curarized animal after artificial respiration has been stopped and the outbursts in the sympathetic are still in phase with the motor discharge in the phrenic"*.

Subsequently, the experimental findings appeared more various and required less simplistic explanations. Koepchen and co-workers (1981) proposed that this second-order sympathetic rhythm could depend on two basic mechanisms: a primary intracentral coupling with the generator of the main cardiovascular respiratory rhythm and a secondary reflex coupling.

For the third-order oscillations Preiss and Polosa (1974) and Polosa (1984) maintained that it is the activity of a central oscillator, in part present at the spinal level (Fernandez de Molina and Perl 1965), which produces the sympathetic rhythm and therefore the Mayer waves.

Mayer waves are known to be increased in amplitude by various manipulations such as hypotensive hemorrhage (Preiss and Polosa 1974), thus suggesting that they might reflect different functional states. As it will be seen, the forthcoming approach is largely based on the fact that in numerous different conditions the increases in sympathetic activity are associated to an enhancement of a third-order rhythm affecting cardiovascular variables.

Computer analysis of cardiovascular signal variability
The activity of sinus node pacemaker cells is under continuous regulation mainly effected by neural mechanisms. The possibility recently offered by computer techniques of quantifying the small spontaneous beat by beat oscillations in cardiovascular variables and in particular in the electrocardiographic RR interval, aroused a growing interest in view of the hypothesis that these rhythmical oscillations could provide some insight into the neural regulatory mechanisms operating in the intact organisms under various real-life conditions.

The application of computationally efficient spectral techniques (Cooley and Tukey 1965) gave the opportunity to assess specifically the possible different rhythmicities hidden in RR interval time series.

Sayers (1973) and his coworkers (Hyndman et al. 1971), for instance, employing the fast Fourier transform (FFT) algorithm, reported the existence in humans of three major components in RR variability that they observed in specific bands of predetermined frequencies around 0.25, 0.10, and 0.03 Hz, respectively; i.e., a respiration-linked component (0.25 Hz) and two others at lower frequencies. Following this pioneering work, several other investigators applied this technique and, in spite of the fact that the heart rate variability signal is not strictly periodical as requested by the deterministic nature of the FFT algorithm, it was proposed by Akselrod et al (1981) that it could be used as a quantitative probe to assess cardiovascular control thus stimulating numerous laboratories, including ours, to enter the game.

As to the neural mechanisms underlying these fluctuations, vagal efferent activity was considered responsible for the higher frequency, i.e., the respiration-linked oscillation of heart rate variability. This conclusion was based on the disappearance of this component after vagotomy performed in experiments on decerebrate cats (Chess et al. 1975), or after muscarinic receptor blockade in conscious dogs (Akselrod et al. 1981) and humans (Selman et al. 1982). Both vagal and sympathetic outflows were considered to determine the lower-frequency components, together with the hypothetical participation of other regulatory mechanisms such as the renin-angiotensin system (Akselrod et al. 1981).

METHODOLOGY

The analysis of heart rate variability (HRV) is usually performed off-line with computerized techniques. After appropriate amplification, filtering and analog-to-digital conversion, various algorithms can be used to assess the duration of individual heart periods, usually considering the peak of the R-wave as the fiducial point. To improve the accuracy of its detection, while keeping the acquisition frequency at 300-500 samples per second, a parabolic interpolation can be implemented in the detection algorithm. The time series of RR intervals that is obtained is stored as the tachogram. It is important to ensure that all beats are of sinus origin, although occasional ectopic beats can be filtered out with a linear interpolation. The presence of frequent arrhythmias can in fact seriously affect the subsequent analysis.

Time domain analysis

Time domain measurements of HRV were initially based on simple statistics, such as the standard deviation (SD) of RR interval variation and its derivatives. This approach, however, does not provide any information on the time structure or periodicity of the data. Additional assessments are represented, e.g., by frequency histograms, geometrical indexes, scattergrams and return maps (Malik and Camm 1995; Task Force 1996).

Frequency domain analysis

The use of spectral analysis implies that the signal series can be represented by a sum of sinusoidal components of different amplitude, frequency and phase values. Various algorithms can be used to assess the number, frequency and amplitude of oscillatory components. The majority of investigators have either relied on FFT algorithm or on autoregressive (AR) modeling. The FFT is easier to implement and is usually employed with *a priori* selection of the number and frequency range of bands of interest. Conversely, AR algorithms can decompose the overall spectrum into single spectral components, using the residual theorem, thus providing automatically the number, central frequency, and associated power of the oscillatory components without the need for *a priori* assumptions (Pagani et al. 1986b; Malliani et al. 1991a; Kamath and Fallen 1993; Task Force 1996). Furthermore AR algorithms have the additional advantage that even with short segments of data (for instance, 200 cycles rather than the more usual 512 cycles) they can provide a reliable and accurate spectral estimation.

The spectrum of Figure 18 contains three components, with frequencies centered at 0.00 Hz (component 1), 0.12 Hz (component 2), and 0.27 Hz (component 3), respectively. The study of the very low frequency (0-0.03 Hz) phenomena (component 1), which might contain relevant information, requires specific methodologies and long periods of uninterrupted data. It is labeled DC or VLF component, according to the emphasis given to the possible presence of either slow trends or very low frequency oscillations. This, component 1, considered either DC or VLF, is not addressed in the present methodology. Components 2 and 3, labeled low frequency (LF) and high frequency (HF) respectively, are evaluated in terms of frequency (hertz in the figures) and amplitude. This amplitude is assessed by the area (i.e., power) of each component; therefore, squared units are used for the absolute value (milliseconds squared in Figure 18). In addition, normalized units (nu) are obtained by dividing the power of a given component by the total variance (from which component 1 has been subtracted) and multiplying by 100 (Figure 18).

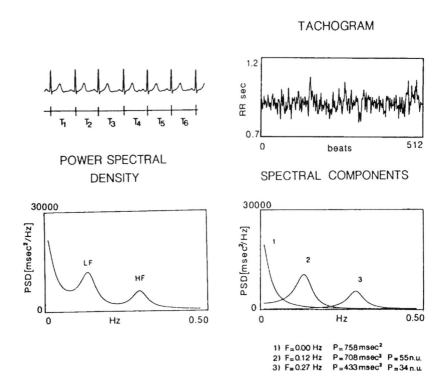

Figure 18: Schematic representation of the method used for the spectral analysis of RR interval variability. From the surface electrocardiogram (top left panel), the program computes the individual RR intervals (T_1-T_6) and stores them in the memory as the tachogram. From the tachogram, power spectral density (PSD) is computed. Two major components, low frequency (LF, component 2) and high frequency (HF, component 3), are usually recognized as well as a large and variable fraction of very slow oscillations (below 0.03 Hz, component 1), which is not considered in the analysis. Note that the computer program automatically recognizes and prints out for each component the central frequency (F) and associated power (P) in absolute ($msec^2$) and normalized units (nu) (see values in lower right panel). In the ordinates of lower panels, PSD units are in $msec^2$/Hz; consequently, their integrated value corresponding to the area (i.e., power, obtained over any given frequency range in Hz) is expressed in $msec^2$. (From Furlan et al. 1990, with permission).

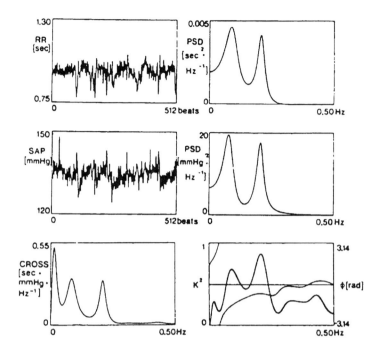

Figure 19: Example of the simultaneous computer analysis of the RR interval and systolic arterial pressure (SAP) variabilities. As explained in the text, after appropriate analog-to-digital conversion of the ECG and arterial pressure signals, the RR interval and SAP series are obtained (top and middle left panels). Then, the corresponding spectra (power spectral density [PSD]) are computed (top and middle right panels). The bottom left panel shows the cross spectrum (Cross); the bottom right panel shows the phase relationship (Φ) and the squared coherence (K^2, curve with two major peaks). (From Pagani et al. 1988b, with permission).

Similarly, the LF/HF ratio can also assess the fractional distribution of power (Pagani et al. 1986b; Malliani et al. 1991a), although, like any ratio, it can emphasize the opposite changes.

This methodology can be applied to any signal such as arterial pressure, respiration or nerve discharge. In the case of simultaneous analysis of RR and systolic arterial pressure (SAP) variabilities, the computer calculates the tachogram (i.e. the series of consecutive RR intervals) as well as the systogram (i.e. the series of maximal systolic values synchronized with each RR interval). As it can be seen in Figure 19, two oscillations, LF and HF components, characterize the power spectra of both RR and SAP variabilities.

As a result the cross spectrum (obtained by frequency transformation of a cross-correlation function) also displays two spectral components. Furthermore a significant coherence (above 0.5) can be detected in Figure 19 (right bottom panel) between the LF and HF spectral components of RR and SAP variability.

In biological terms, this indicates that the two rhythms are significantly correlated within the same frequency. As to the phase, its negative values indicate, according to convention, that RR lags behind SAP (Baselli et al. 1986).

A recursive version of this methodology permits the analysis of recordings over a 24-hour period. Like the HF respiratory component, LF oscillation does not have a fixed period, and its central frequency can vary considerably (from 0.04 to 0.13 Hz) (Pagani et al. 1988b; Furlan et al. 1990). Therefore, the initial convention of subdividing the low part of the spectrum into two preselected bands with a cutoff frequency of 0.07 Hz (Parati et al. 1990) contained within the range of LF component appears by now unjustified (Malliani et al. 1991a; Fagard et al. 1998).

Time-variant analysis

More recent approaches attempted to analyze the time development of frequency components thus providing information in both time and frequency domain. However, only relatively fast transients can be detected with these approaches that include the smoothed pseudo-Wigner-Ville transformation (SPWVT) and the time-variant autoregressive approach. Examples will be provided subsequently in the book.

PHYSIOLOGICAL STUDIES

The core hypothesis of the proposed approach is that the sympathovagal balance, viewed as a reciprocal relation, can on the whole be explored in the frequency domain. I shall review data that support the assumptions that 1) the respiratory rhythm of heart period variability, defined as HF spectral component, is a marker of vagal modulation; 2) the rhythm corresponding to vasomotor waves and present in heart period and arterial pressure variabilities, defined as LF component, is a marker of sympathetic modulation; and 3) a reciprocal relation exists between these two rhythms that is similar to that characterizing the sympathovagal balance.

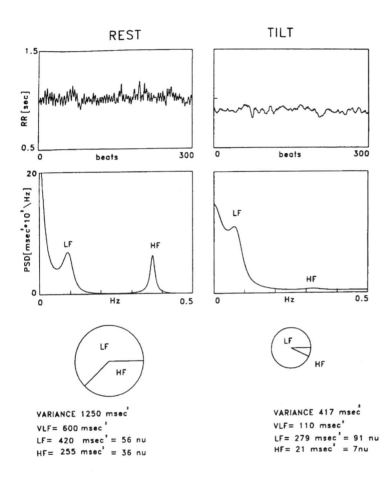

Figure 20: Spectral analysis of HRV in a young subject at rest and during 90° tilt. The RR interval time series (i.e., tachograms) are illustrated in the top panels. The middle panels contain the autospectra (PSD = power spectral density) which indicate the presence of two major components (LF = low frequency; HF = high frequency). During tilt, the LF component becomes largely predominant. In this example the total power (i.e. variance) is markedly reduced during tilt and consequently LF and HF powers are both decreased when expressed in absolute units. The use of normalized units (nu) clearly indicates the altered relation between LF and HF during tilt as represented by the pie charts which show the relative distribution together with the absolute power of the two components represented by the area. (From Malliani et al. 1997a, with permission).

The order I shall follow in the description of the most relevant observations made so far is only partially respectful of the temporal sequence of their acquisitions, but is rather focused on the intent to provide a simple key to interpret this complex matter.

Human studies
Effects of maneuvers enhancing sympathetic activity
Passive tilt or, more simply, standing up is invariably accompanied in healthy adolescents or adults by a relative increase in the LF and decrease in the HF component of RR variability (Figure 20).

This was the first physiological maneuver that we adopted in our studies (Brovelli et al. 1983) in order to shift sympathovagal balance towards sympathetic excitation. The constant and drastic change in spectral profile was, however, often accompanied by a marked decrease in total power (corresponding to variance). Our hypothesis has been, since the very beginning, that the most relevant information concerning sympathovagal balance was likely to be contained in the fractional distribution of power, independently of the absolute values of variance and of the VLF component.

Thus we resorted to a normalization procedure already alluded to in the METHODOLOGY section. It has only to be further specified that usually the sum of LFnu and HFnu (Figures 18 and 20) is less than 100 because of the frequent presence of small noise components.

The normalization procedure has indeed proved crucial to the interpretation of data. In fact, when sympathetic excitation is accompanied by a reduction of variance, the absolute values of LF undergo contrasting influences – as they tend to be decreased by the reduction of variance but also tend to be increased by the greater concentration of power in the LF component, as reflected by its constant rise in nu. Conversely, the HF component is decreased during tilt in both absolute and normalized units.

However, the heuristic value of this conceptual approach, coupling one rhythm (LF) with sympathetic and one rhythm (HF) with vagal modulation, requires sound proofs before being evident.

The first was obtained during a study (Montano et al. 1994) in which we investigated the capability of power spectrum analysis of HRV to assess the changes in sympathovagal balance during graded orthostatic tilt. In our hypothesis, the sympathetic excitation and the vagal withdrawal characterizing the orthostatic position were conceived as the endpoint in a continuum of intermediate changes paralleling the progression of the stimulus. Healthy volunteers were thus subjected to a series of passive head-up tilt steps randomly chosen among the following angles: 15°, 30°, 45°, 60°, and 90°. As already reported (Pagani et al. 1986b; Lipsitz et al. 1990), age was significantly correlated to variance and to the absolute values in msec^2 of LF and HF components.

A strong correlation was found between the degree of tilt incline and LF and HF components expressed in nu (r = 0.78 and –0.70, p < 0.001, respectively) (Figure 21).

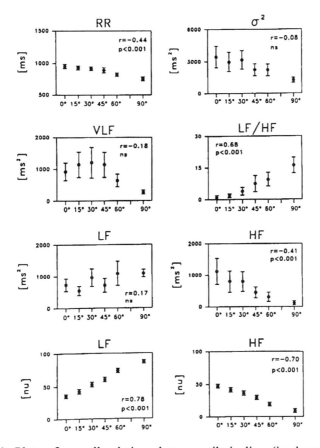

Figure 21: Plots of overall relations between tilt incline (in degrees) and measures of RR interval variability. σ^2 indicates variance; VLF, very low frequency; LF, low frequency; HF, high frequency; LF/HF=ratio of low frequency to high frequency; nu, normalized units; and r, Spearman's correlation coefficient. (From Montano et al. 1994, with permission).

When LF was expressed in absolute units, no significant correlation was found as well as with variance, while a significant albeit smaller correlation was detected with RR and HF in absolute units (r = -0.44 and -0.41, p < 0.001, respectively). A strong correlation was present with LF/HF ratio (r = 0.68, p < 0.001). Hence, on similar very high probability grounds, this study appears to legitimize a sort of circling conclusion. On one side, the hypothesis that sympathetic excitation and vagal withdrawal progress in a continuum seems reinforced, while on the other side, the conclusion seems supported *a fortiori* that this methodology, without artificially separating the influence of either neural outflow, can reveal with unprecedented efficacy some aspects of neural regulation.

Similar findings were obtained by Bootsma et al. (1994).

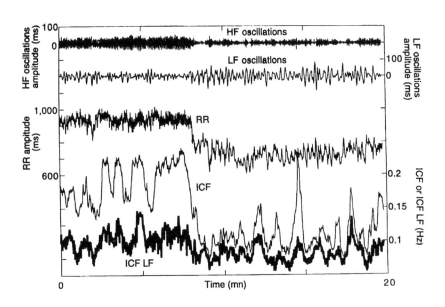

Figure 22: Time-frequency analysis of heart rate variability of a healthy subject in supine position followed by passive tilt at 90°. Metronome breathing at 0.25 Hz. Amplitude of oscillations was obtained by finite impulse response filtering. Top to bottom: amplitude HF and LF (ms), RR interval (ms), and instant center frequency (in Hz) of whole spectral power (ICF) and of LF (ICF LF). Tilt between 7 and 8 minutes. (Modified from Jasson et al. 1997, with permission).

The second proof was obtained by Jasson et al. (1997) utilizing an algorithm (smoothed pseudo-Wigner-Ville transformation) which is capable, as anticipated in the METHODOLOGY section, of detecting transients and of displaying a frequency domain analysis over time (Figure 22). In spite of its technical complexity, the biological interpretation of this Figure is quite simple. In the upper two tracings the HF and LF oscillations can be appreciated in both their frequency and amplitude characteristics. The third tracing is the usual tachogram (RR), while the fourth tracing represents the instant center frequency (ICF) of the whole spectrum, i.e. the median frequency of the whole power distribution. The bottom tracing is a similar instant center frequency calculated for the LF component (ICF LF). These recordings were obtained from a normal subject who, after an initial period in a resting horizontal position, was passively tilted to an upright position at 90° (between the 7th and 8th minute). During tilt the following simultaneous changes occurred and were maintained throughout its duration: the amplitude of HF decreased, that of LF increased, heart period also decreased indicating a tachycardia response, ICF underwent a decrease indicating that spectral power was redistributed towards the lower frequencies. In short, all the changes indicated a shift in sympathovagal balance towards sympathetic excitation and vagal inhibition.

Thus the push-pull organization of LF and HF oscillations is self-evident and is independent of a normalization procedure. This aspect is important as the use of normalized units has been criticized (Eckberg 1997) in view of their inherent mathematical simplicity: instead I think that this simplicity adequately reflects a basic biological strategy of antagonistic subsystems (Malliani et al. 1998).

The simultaneous recording of muscle sympathetic nerve activity (MSNA), however, was going to furnish an additional crucial proof of the validity of the whole approach.

In a study on healthy volunteers, Pagani et al (1997) reported the effects of graded changes in arterial pressure induced by infusion of nitroprusside or phenylephrine, i.e. the effects of graded deactivations or stimulations of arterial baroreflexogenic areas. The sympathetic excitation induced by nitroprusside was accompanied not only by an increase in LFnu component of RR and SAP variabilities (as already observed during tilt by Pagani et al. 1986b) but also by a clear increase in LFnu component of MSNA (Figure 23, left panels). As a crucial detail, a tight average correlation was found between the LFnu component of RR variability and the LFnu component of muscle sympathetic nerve activity (MSNA).

Hence, the general phenomenon was that during sympathetic excitation, in normal humans, there was a predominance of the coherent LF oscillations present in heart period, arterial pressure and MSNA.

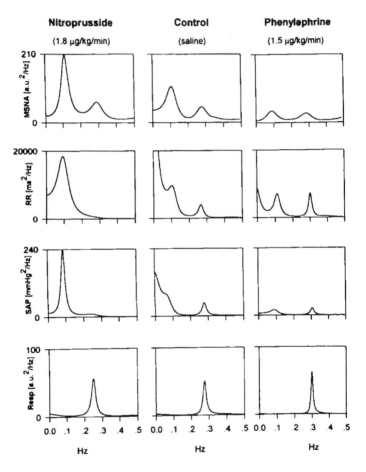

Figure 23: Power spectra of MSNA, RR interval, SAP variabilities, and respiration (Resp) in a single subject during infusions of saline (Control), nitroprusside, and phenylephrine. During sympathetic activation induced by nitroprusside (left), the LF component of neural and cardiovascular variability signals predominates relative to the HF component. Conversely, during sympathetic inhibition and vagal activation induced by phenylephrine (right), there is an increase of the HF component relative to the LF component. a.u. indicates arbitrary units. (From Pagani et al. 1997, with permission).

Although a great deal of specificity exists in the various contingents of sympathetic outflow and, consequently, the functional characteristics of MSNA recorded from the leg cannot be simply ascribed to the sympathetic activity directed to the heart, baroreflex deactivation is known to lead to a widely distributed reflex sympathetic excitation. This study seems to confirm this latter principle.

However the indisputable proof of the pragmatic value of both the concept of sympathovagal balance and of the corollary normalization procedure has been furnished by a study (Malliani et al. 1997b) the protocol of which included 350 healthy subjects from whom ECG and respiratory recordings were obtained in controlled laboratory conditions. Each subject was studied in both supine and upright positions. Individual data were ordered consecutively in their historical sequence and, subsequently, odd and even rank positions were assigned respectively to a Training or Test set, respectively. Hence, Training and Test sets each held 350 patterns characterized by 10 power spectrum variables belonging to 175 subjects studied in both supine and upright positions. The variables were the following: RR mean, variance, VLF $msec^2$, LF Hz, LF $msec^2$, LFnu, HF Hz, HF $msec^2$, HF nu, LF/HF ratio. The features related to both postures were considered as independent.

A forecasting linear method concentrated the information distributed in the various spectral variables into a normalized activation index (AI) (ranging from −1 for supine to +1 for upright posture). During the Training set the algorithm had to match the target, i.e. the posture, which was classified by the experimenter, with the information that could be extracted from the interaction of the variables of interest. A pattern was correctly discriminated when the supine position corresponded to an AI between 0 and −1 and the upright position to an AI between 0 and +1. During the Test set, as well, a negative value of the AI was intended to recognize the supine and a positive value the upright position. Such a blind forecasting on the Test set was capable of correctly assigning 83.4% (146 of 175) of features to group supine and 86.3% (151 of 175) to group upright, when 10 variables were evaluated simultaneously. Three variables (RR, LFnu and HFnu) were found to hold almost all the information content, and could recognize an overall 84% patterns, with a similarly good performance in both supine and upright groups (Figure 24). When one of these three variables was not considered, the forecasting provided inconsistent results.

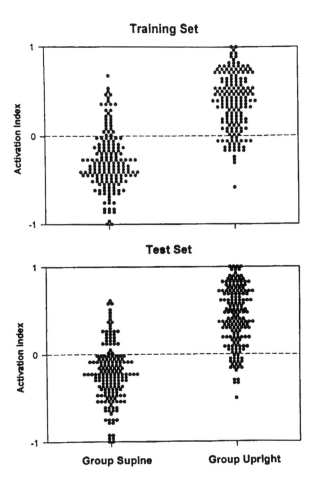

Figure 24: Activation Index (AI) of each individual feature belonging either to the Training or Test set. Negative Als were normalized, for supine posture, between zero and –1, and positive Als were normalized, for upright posture, between zero and +1. Three variables (RR, LFnu, HFnu) were used for discrimination and recognition rates. In the Test set, 33 features were unrecognized in the supine group and 23 in the upright group, whereas all others were correctly assigned. (From Malliani et al. 1997b, with permission).

Supine and upright postures, as an example of well-reproducible physiological conditions, are known to engender distinct levels of sympathetic and vagal activity and hence of sympathovagal balance. It was reported, for the first time, that a physiological non invasive recording, such as the ECG contains an intrinsic information that can be used to recognize, individual by individual, the two different autonomic profiles related to posture. In addition to RR interval, the most powerful variables for both discrimination and recognition rates appeared to be LFnu and HFnu, according to our hypothesis.

In the experiments in which the sympathetic excitation was obtained either during upright position or arterial hypotension, it is likely that arterial baroreflexes were playing a critical role.

However a sympathetic excitation can also be obtained independently of baroreflex mechanisms as in the case of mental activity or physical exercise. Mental stress induced by arithmetic calculation is accompanied by a shift of sympathovagal balance, a reduction in total power, an increase in LFnu and a decrease in HFnu of RR variability (Pagani et al. 1989, 1991).

Physical exercise, overwhelming baroreflex restraint, also increases sympathetic activity and is associated with additional factors such as enhanced respiratory activity, and increased non stationarity.

In humans, heart rate may vary from ~50 beats/min at rest to ~200 beats/min during maximal exercise, corresponding to intervals ranging between 1,200 and 300 ms. Its standard deviation is about one order of magnitude less, ranging in short-term laboratory recordings from ~50 msec at rest to ~6 msec during extreme tachycardia. Hence, a drastically reduced HRV signal (i.e. variance) contributes to a difficult analysis. However, Pagani et al (1988b) described, for mild levels of exercise, a clear predominance of the LF component in RR variability.

Quite recently Iellamo et al (1999) reported a marked shift of sympathovagal balance towards sympathetic excitation during hypertension and tachycardia accompanying one leg static exercise, in well acceptable stationary conditions.

During heavier exercise the increases in nonstationarity and nonlinearity require specific algorithms such as Coarse Graining Spectral Analysis (Yamamoto et al. 1991) which seems capable of assessing the progressive changes in autonomic modulation.

Systolic arterial pressure variability
The study of SAP variability has indicated that LF component is invariably increased during tilt (Pagani et al. 1986b) and sympathetic activation obtained with baroreceptor deactivation (Figure 23, left panels). In the case of LF_{SAP} component a normalization procedure is not necessary in order to appreciate this enhancement because arterial pressure variance does not decrease but rather increases during

sympathetic excitation induced by tilt. However, the use of normalized units provides similar findings.

Concerning physical exercise, the study of arterial pressure variability requires particular recording techniques in order to reduce the mechanical artifacts. Thus we applied a microminiature Millar catheter-tip pressure transducer to the Holter recording of ambulatory arterial pressure (Pagani et al. 1986a). In this way it was possible to detect an increase in LF component of systolic arterial pressure during various degrees of physical exercise (Furlan et al. 1987; Rimoldi et al. 1992; Piazza et al. 1995). On the whole, LF_{SAP} was proposed as a marker of sympathetic modulation of vasomotor activity.

It might be interesting to further specify that during treadmill exercise (Piazza et al. 1995) a very high frequency component (0.94 Hz) was evident in arterial pressure power spectrum, corresponding to the frequency of 112 foot impacts per minute. In the high-fidelity recordings this mechanical event was however quite smaller when compared to the 70-80 mmHg oscillations recorded with a saline-filled catheter, leading to the description of a "beat" phenomenon (Palatini et al. 1989).

Effects of maneuvers enhancing vagal activity

Controlled respiration at frequencies within the resting physiological range (Kitney et al. 1982) provides a convenient tool to enhance the vagal modulation of heart period. The power of the HF component becomes predominant at rest during metronome breathing – in the study by Pagani et al (1986b) the LF/HF ratio was significantly reduced from 2.5 to 0.7. Furthermore, during controlled respiration, increases in the LF component and LF/HF ratio induced by tilt were markedly blunted in regard to those obtained during spontaneous respiration (Pagani et al. 1986b).

When the frequency of controlled breathing is decreased enough to approach LF rhythm, the two components merge into one more powerful oscillation, the so-called "entrainment" (Kitney et al. 1982; Malliani et al. 1991a). In laboratory experiments, by monitoring respiratory movements, it should always be ascertained that their spontaneous frequency does not correspond to LF, discarding the cases in which this occurs. On the other hand the experiments that have been performed under controlled respiration in the broad range of 0.20 to 0.30 Hz were all likely to be characterized by a sympathovagal balance shifted in favor of the vagal component (Pomeranz et al. 1985; Cooke et al. 1999).

Accordingly, in a recent study by Cooke et al (1999) controlled respiration at 12 breaths per min (0.2 Hz) was accompanied during graded tilt by a blunted change in spectral profile with an HF component still prevailing on the LF component when the subjects were inclined to 80°. Moreover, at the end of tilting maneuver, end-tidal CO_2 concentrations were reduced by 22%.

It is obvious that controlled respiration does not correspond to physiological conditions especially when associated with a disturbance of blood gases. In addition Cooke et al (1999) when measuring LF_{RR} eluded the use and failed to mention the very existence of a normalization procedure, which would have led to data not too dissimilar from ours (Pagani et al. 1997), not quoted, concluding instead: *"our data provide a strong argument against use of low-frequency of R-R interval spectral power as a non-invasive index of sympathetic activity"*. This was exactly what had been previously found by Montano et al (1994), also unquoted, when the degree of tilt was assessed by LF_{RR} in absolute units (Figure 21).

Baroreceptor stimulation obtained, e.g., with pressor drugs is also capable of shifting the sympathovagal balance towards vagal predominance (Figure 23, right panels). Rotation or cold stimulation of the face represent other maneuvers capable of inducing a prevalence of HF component (Malliani et al. 1994b)

Finally, the experiments by Tougas et al (1997) should be quoted as they indicated that both electrical and mechanical oesophageal stimulation increased the HF component of RR variability while simultaneously decreasing the LF component.

Continuous 24-hour analysis

Initial observations (Pagani et al. 1985a) with spectral analysis clearly indicated the possibility of assessing the circadian oscillations of the sympathovagal balance. When LF was analyzed in nu over the 24-hour period (Furlan et al. 1990; Guzzetti et al. 1991a; Malliani et al. 1991a; Bernardi et al. 1992; Lombardi et al. 1992) it displayed a clear circadian pattern (Figure 25) with a marked nocturnal decrease corresponding to the well-known reduction of sympathetic activity. These changes were mirrored by simultaneous increases in HF component, as an expression of the enhanced vagal activity accompanying the largest portion of sleep. The LF component could

86

instead appear unchanged, or even increased during the night, if expressed in absolute units, in parallel with the nocturnal rise of variance leading to the unwarranted conclusion that *"24 hour LF power is primarily parasympathetically and not sympathetically mediated"* (Goldsmith et al. 1992). But, as we have already questioned (Pagani et al. 1993), *"at which point and on which grounds quantity (i.e., length of data) would invert quality (i.e., shifting from sympathetic into parasympathetic modulation)?"*

Furthermore, the circadian oscillation of the LF component that we have described was not observed in a study (Parati et al. 1990) in which this component was subdivided into two predetermined bands of interest with a cutoff frequency of 0.07 Hz, and the heart period was derived from ambulatory pressure recordings performed with a system of narrow frequency response. This obviously stresses the importance of an adequate spectral methodology.

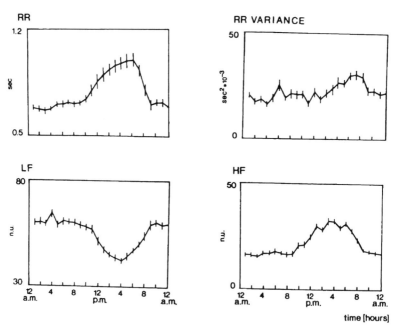

Figure 25: Plots of average hourly values of RR interval, of its variance (in absolute units), and LF and HF components (in normalized units) during 24 hours in a group of nonhospitalized subjects free to move. (From Furlan et al. 1990, with permission).

Finally, continuous 24-hour analysis of SAP variability (Furlan et al. 1990) indicated that the LF component of SAP variability, obtained from ambulant subjects with a high-fidelity recording system, increased abruptly upon awakening, while the patients were still in bed, and remained elevated throughout the day. Physical activity induced further increases in the LF component of SAP variability, which, conversely, underwent a marked reduction during the night.

This abrupt surge of sympathetic activity in the early morning or upon awakening is obviously highly suspected of being involved as a trigger mechanism in the increased incidence of acute cardiovascular events occurring during the same morning hours (Muller et al. 1989)

Animal studies

The possibility of applying the same methodology to human subjects and to experimental animals, employing both non invasive and invasive signal recordings, has provided a notable interaction of notions acquired during quite different experimental conditions.

A dominant role of the vagi in determining the HF component of RR variability was inferred from experiments in acute decerebrate cats (Chess et al. 1975) and conscious dogs (Akselrod et al. 1981, 1985; Rimoldi et al. 1990), describing the effects of vagotomy and muscarinic receptor blockade.

Furthermore, Rimoldi et al (1990) reported that in resting conscious dogs characterized by a marked HF predominance (Figure 26) resulting from high vagal tone (Brown et al. 1989), a small LF component was always present in SAP variability but only in 50% of the cases in RR variability. However, an important finding was that whenever sympathetic excitation occurred, such as during baroreceptor unloading with nitroglycerin infusion, transient coronary artery occlusion, or physical exercise, a significant increase in LF was observed (Figure 26).

The role played by baroreceptive mechanisms in these various experimental conditions was probably different because arterial pressure was reduced by nitroglycerin infusion, unchanged during myocardial ischemia, and increased with exercise. Therefore, LF component should not be considered a specific reflection of a baroreflex compensatory response (Appel et al. 1989) but rather a general marker of sympathetic excitation, regardless of its mechanism.

During muscarinic receptor blockade (Rimoldi et al. 1990), which drastically reduced total RR variance, all of the remaining power in control conditions and during baroreceptor unloading was concentrated in the LF region, in accordance with the sympathetic predominance induced by the drug.

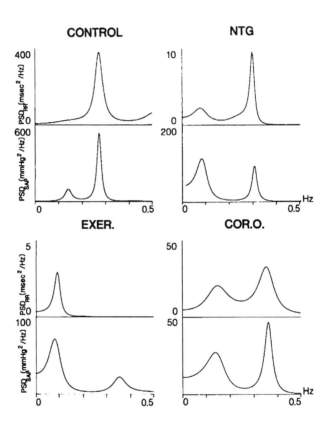

Figure 26: Spectral analysis of RR interval (upper tracings in each panel) and SAP (lower tracings in each panel) variabilities in conscious dogs at rest (CONTROL) and during experimental maneuvers leading to a sympathetic predominance (i.e., nitroglycerin infusion (NTG), treadmill exercise (EXER.), and transient acute coronary artery occlusion (COR.O.). Note at control the presence of a single major HF component in the RR interval autospectrum; in SAP, a smaller LF component is also evident. During sympathetic activation, spectral distribution is altered in favor of LF; simultaneously, a drastic reduction in RR variance occurs (notice different scales on ordinates). PSD, power spectral density. (From Malliani et al. 1991a, with permission).

Finally, after chronic bilateral stellectomy producing cardiac sympathetic denervation, baroreceptor unloading no longer induced an increase in the LF component of RR variability. On the contrary, the increase in the LF component of SAP variability was still present.

It was inferred that in RR variability, HF was mainly mediated by vagal mechanisms, whereas the sympathetic outflow appeared essential to the LF increases. Furthermore, the importance of neural mechanisms in mediating LF and HF of RR variability and LF of SAP variability was proven by their disappearance during ganglionic transmission blockade, obtained with intravenous infusion of trimethaphan (Rimoldi et al. 1990).

Experiments on acute decerebrate cats, artificially ventilated, in which ECG, arterial pressure and thoracic sympathetic preganglionic activity were recorded, furnished the first evidence of a central reciprocal relation between LF and HF rhythms (Montano et al. 1992).

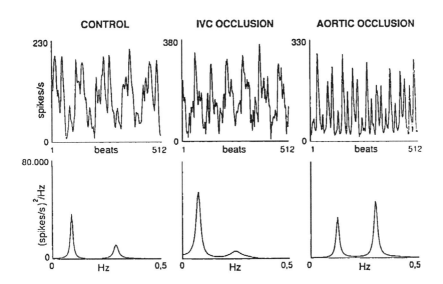

Figure 27: Spectral analysis of SND during control inferior vena cava (IVC) and aortic occlusion. The time series of neural discharge is presented in the top panels, the autospectra in the lower panels. Two distinct spectral components at LF and HF are evident in control conditions. A markedly predominant LF component is present during IVC occlusion, while two well-defined components of similar magnitude are evident during aortic constriction. Data are from a decerebrate cat. (From Montano et al. 1992, with permission).

For instance, it was observed (Figure 27) that a sympathetic excitation (obtained with a reduction in arterial pressure during inferior vena cava occlusion) modified the relationship between the LF and HF components present in the sympathetic discharge, increasing LF predominance. Conversely, during sympathetic inhibition (obtained with baroreceptor stimulation during aortic occlusion) the relationship was clearly shifted towards HF predominance. The LF and HF components of RR variability underwent similar changes.

Finally, a significant and positive correlation was found between the changes in the sympathetic efferent discharge and the amplitude of LF component of either RR interval or sympathetic discharge variabilities.

Smaller animals with faster heart rate have a reduced HRV from which, however, LF and HF components – coherent with similar components present in SAP variability – can be detected with FFT (Japundzic et al.1990), autoregressive (Rubini et al. 1993) or more peculiar algorithms (Carré et al. 1994). Their frequencies in Hz are remarkably higher (LF around 0.45 Hz and HF around 1.35 Hz) due to the higher heart rate but they correspond to usual values (LF around 0.1 and HF around 0.25) when considered in cycles/cardiac beat (Rubini et al. 1993). This discloses an issue that deserves a short comment.

With autoregressive algorithms the duration of the periodical phenomena in the variability signal is measured as a function of cardiac beats, rather than seconds. As an example, a four-beat periodical component is represented with a frequency of 1:4, i.e., 0.25 cycle/beat. However, this frequency is easily converted into hertz equivalents (Hz Eq) by dividing it by the average RR interval length. For instance, if the average RR length is 1000 msec, this corresponds to 0.25 Hz Eq. In our first extensive article (Pagani et al. 1986b), both units (c/b and Hz Eq) were indicated, whereas subsequently, according to common convention, only Hz have been used. In general it appears obvious that the heart period might represent a more essential variable for the organization of cardiovascular rhythmicity than an external clock.

The use of small animals appears particularly important for future developments. For instance, Mansier et al (1996b) found that in transgenic mice, with a specific eightfold atrial overexpression of human β_1-adrenoceptor, HRV was nearly suppressed, while heart rate was unchanged. This clearly indicated that HR and HRV provide quite different information.

There are, however, pathophysiological problems that have been until now better addressed with more traditional experimental models. It is the case, for instance, of experiments carried out in conscious dogs with heart failure induced by rapid ventricular pacing (Eaton et al. 1995; Ishise et al. 1998). A decline in ventricular contractility and a progression in diastolic dysfunction were accompanied by a shift of sympathovagal balance towards sympathetic predominance, as assessed by HRV spectral analysis.

Rimoldi et al (1990) could observe in conscious dogs the profound change in autonomic profile accompanying a transient coronary artery occlusion in the absence of behavioral changes suggesting the presence of pain (Figures 26 and 28).

These experiments, in addition to those by Pagani et al (1985b), also documented in conscious animals the occurrence of a cardiocardiac sympathetic reflex, that previously could only have been found in acute experimental conditions.

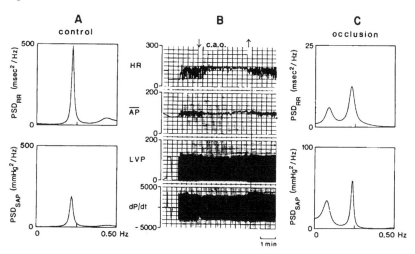

Figure 28: Effects of a transient, non-hypotensive, coronary artery occlusion (c.a.o. between arrows, *B*) on RR and systolic arterial pressure (SAP) variabilities power spectral density (PSD) in a conscious dog. Note that during occlusion (*C*) there is a reduction in variance from control (*A*) (see also the tachogram in *B*), together with appearance of a large LF component in both RR and SAP power spectrum, as a reflection of increase in sympathetic efferent activity. LVP: left ventricular pressure; dP/dt: rate of change of left ventricular pressure. (From Rimoldi et al. 1990, with permission).

Pharmacological blockades and neural lesions

The observations by Selman et al (1982) documented that atropine administration was capable of practically abolishing the respiratory component of RR variability. This finding was corroborated by the study of Pomeranz et al (1985). On the basis of these experiments as well as the already quoted animal studies, the relation between vagal activity and HF component of RR variability has become generally accepted.

However, it is my opinion that these observations do not imply at all a *pure* vagal nature of HF component, as maintained by most authors. I consider this subtractive reasoning simply incapable of detecting the complex nature of HF component (Malliani 1995). An HF component is clearly present in sympathetic nerve efferent discharge (Figure 23 and 27) and the hypothesis appears almost deprived of biological common sense that the influence of HF sympathetic rhythm is practically abolished by the low-pass filter properties of sympathetic transmission (Appel et al. 1989). It is hard to find even one single acceptable proof for the ineffectual nature of an established biological phenomenon.

It is interesting to point out that Hedman et al (1995) have observed in anesthetized dogs that an increased sympathetic activity directed to the heart is capable of reducing the HF component of HRV. Still in this perspective, the remarkable experiments by Kawada et al (1996, 1997) have clearly indicated that simultaneous vagal and sympathetic excitations increase the heart rate responses bidirectionally, thus extending the dynamic range of neural regulation, in line with the concept of accentuated antagonism (Levy 1971).

The disagreement in the literature regarding the interpretation of the LF component is much more substantial.

In the same study by Pomeranz et al (1985) intravenous administration of atropine in supine patients under controlled respiration was also capable of reducing the LF component by 84%; it was concluded that, in this position, the LF component is mediated entirely by the parasympathetic system. However, calculations of LF/HF ratio from their average published data suggest that this ratio (~0.5, i.e., a value very close to the ~0.7 found by Pagani et al (1986b) with autoregressive algorithms in subjects under controlled respiration) was increased by muscarinic receptor blockade to ~1, thus indicating a shift in power distribution in favor of LF. In short, in our opinion the data by Pomeranz et al (1985) could be interpreted in a quite different manner: in conditions of vagal predominance induced by metronome breathing, atropine induces a sympathetic predominance as revealed by the LF/HF ratio. Obviously these data would probably have been clearer if the subjects were breathing spontaneously and if spectral components were evaluated in normalized units.

In terms of subtractive reasoning, the papers by Inoue et al (1990, 1991) were of crucial importance. These authors reported that the LF component was absent in the RR variability spectrum of six quadriplegic patients (Inoue et al. 1990) and in the SAP variability spectrum of seven similar patients (Inoue et al. 1991). The interpretation of these findings was that the absence of an LF component in RR and SAP variability spectra was likely to depend upon the interruption at the spinal level of those pathways connecting supraspinal centers, where these rhythms were considered to originate, with spinal sympathetic outflow.

However, the reality turned out to be more complex. In a subsequent study we examined the heart period and SAP variabilities in 15 chronic, neurologically complete, quadriplegic patients during control conditions, head-up tilt and controlled respiration (Guzzetti et al. 1994a). In seven of these patients no LF component was present in resting conditions, in RR and SAP variabilities, thus confirming the data by Inoue et al (1990, 1991). Vice versa, in six quadriplegic patients an LF component was clearly detectable in the spectrum of both variability signals, although it was reduced in absolute and normalized units if compared with control subjects. In the two remaining patients, an LF component was present in the spectrum of RR variability only. During tilt, in three of the four patients presenting an adequate HR response (i.e., a tachycardia of at least 10%) a paradoxical LF response was found as this component became no longer detectable in either spectra. Furthermore, the six patients who presented an LF component in both RR and SAP variabilities maintained it during controlled respiration. Finally, in five patients, two recording sessions were performed with a lapse of about 6 months between them. During the second recording, the LFnu component of RR variability appeared markedly increased in three of the four patients in whom this component was already detectable, and became evident in the remaining patient. The LF component of SAP variability spectrum underwent similar changes. Variance also tended to increase during the second recording, although changes were not significant.

These findings could be explained by two opposite hypotheses. The LF component could be mediated at rest by vagal mechanisms, and its disappearance during tilt, as well as the tachycardia response, could reflect a vagal withdrawal (Koh et al. 1994). However, within this hypothesis it is surprising that LF was not present in all patients studied a few months after the lesion, when vagal tone seems to predominate (Mathias and Frankel 1988); on the contrary, it appeared to increase with time, as revealed by the repeated recordings. Furthermore, two quadriplegic patients were characterized by an LF component only in the RR variability spectrum. Thus LF was unlikely to represent an exclusive HR baroreflex vagal response to vasomotor waves as suggested by Appel et al (1989) and Koh et al (1994).

Conversely, the LF component in RR and SAP variabilities could signal the development of a spinal rhythmicity, increasing with time and influencing the various levels of sympathetic outflow distributed to the heart and peripheral vessels. However, the puzzling finding within this second hypothesis corresponds to the LF decrease or disappearance with tilt. Our satellite hypothesis is the following: the reductions in venous return and cardiac dimensions that accompany a tilting maneuver are likely to decrease the discharge of the cardiovascular thoracic sympathetic afferent fibers and thereby the reflex activity of the sympathetic outflow. On the contrary, controlled respiration in quadriplegic patients might provide a way to activate simultaneously vagal pulmonary afferents and those cardiovascular vagal and sympathetic afferent fibers highly sensitive to volume changes. Hence, both vagovagal and sympathosympathetic circuits might be excited, each with its prevailing rhythm, with no possibility for a reciprocal relationship due to the interruption of neural linking pathways. And, in fact, some quadriplegic patients (Guzzetti et al. 1994a) developed or maintained unchanged an LF component in RR and SAP variability spectra during controlled respiration, while normal subjects are usually characterized by a reduction of LF component under these conditions (Pagani et al. 1986b).

An additional intriguing finding, however, in terms of subtractive reasoning, deals with the effects of β-adrenergic receptor blockade on RR variability power spectrum (Pagani et al. 1986b).

Acute propranolol administration in healthy subjects significantly increased RR interval variance but normalized autospectral components in resting conditions were not modified significantly.

During tilt, there was a significantly smaller increase in LFnu component, compared with the same subjects before blockade.

Chronic β-blockade also increased the variance. However significant changes were observed in the resting autospectra: LF was smaller, HF greater and hence LF/HF ratio was reduced. During tilt, the LFnu component was reduced and HFnu component was increased, compared with similar conditions before blockade. Thus, with chronic β-adrenergic receptor blockade, LF/HF ratio increased during tilt to only 3.80±0.80 which was smaller than that observed in the same young subjects (20-30 years) before β-blockade (20.8±3.5).

Hence, while it is obvious that β-adrenergic receptor blockade shifted sympathovagal balance towards vagal predominance, a stronger quantitative action might also have been expected. This phenomenon might partly depend on the incompleteness of a pharmacological blockade in the clinical setting. On the other hand it is difficult to attribute to vagal withdrawal the residual increase in LF during tilt. In fact we still ignore the characteristics of synaptic transmission necessary to induce an oscillatory modulation with respect to usual stimulus-response curves.

Interestingly, it was reported (Lazzeri et al. 1998) that clonidine, a centrally acting inhibitor of sympathetic activity (Hoffman and Leskowitz 1996) reduced LFnu and LF/HF of HRV in healthy subjects. As expected, α-adrenergic receptor blockade drastically reduced LF component of SAP variability (Japundzic et al. 1990; Rubini et al. 1993) or abolished its increase during exercise (Rimoldi et al. 1992)

Modeling approaches

Various models of the complex instantaneous relationship between heart rate and arterial pressure have been proposed (DeBoer, 1985; DeBoer et al. 1986). Usually, the slope of the linear regression of the heart period, as a function of systolic arterial pressure (RR/SAP) plotted during the pressor rise produced by the intravenous injection of a pressor agent such as phenylephrine, is taken as a measure of the gain of the baroreflex control of heart rate (Smyth et al. 1969).

Clinically, this approach modeled as an open loop, in spite of its simplifications, has provided a very useful tool. Recently it has been extended to furnish a more frequent but far from continuous estimate of the gain of baroreflex mechanisms over periods of 24h (Bertinieri et al. 1988; Legramante et al. 1999) as seen in *Chapter 1*. Yet, it does not take into account the fact that changes in heart period can also induce variations in stroke volume, and hence in systolic arterial pressure.

When the circulation is modeled as a closed-loop coupling between heart period and arterial pressure, the transfer function between SAP and RR variabilities describes the neural links between these two signals, while considering also the simultaneous mechanical coupling between RR and SAP (Akselrod et al. 1985). All perturbations, such as respiration, that are not explicitly accounted for by this model are labeled as noise external to the loop.

In Figure 29, the two transfer functions H_{st} and H_{ts} describe the simultaneous effect of heart period (tachogram, t) on systogram (s) and of systogram on tachogram, respectively.

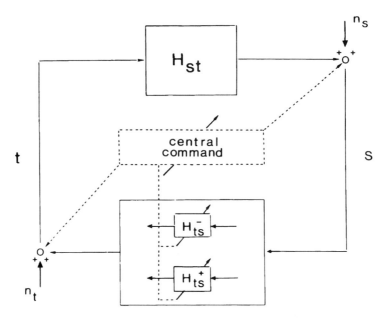

Figure 29: Schematic representation of the closed loop model of the relationship between tachogram (t) and systogram (s). In this scheme the neural block contains both negative (H_{ts}^-) and positive (H_{ts}^+) feedback mechanisms. Thus, the gain of transfer function depends on the complex interaction between these functional components and the central command. (From Pagani et al. 1988b, with permission).

While the effect of tachogram on systogram (H_{st}), is mainly mechanical (upper box), the effect of systogram on tachogram (H_{ts}) is largely mediated by neural reflexes including both *negative and positive feedback* mechanisms (lower box).

H's are generally complex operators (commonly expressed under the form of gain and phase) that are functions of frequency. Two noises, n_t and n_s, are also indicated to describe the external inputs to the system, such as mechanical disturbances, respiration, and small adjustments by *central command*, to take into account all the possible sources that can cause variability of the *t* or *s* signal independently of *s* or *t*, respectively.

This model provides a way of computing an index of the overall gain of this neural interaction (i.e., the relationship between heart period and arterial pressure variabilities) by spectral and cross-spectral analysis. As shown in Figure 19, both tachogram and systogram variabilities contain, at rest, two major components, respectively LF and HF. If, as in the case of Figure 19, the coherence function between these two variabilities is high (i.e., > 0.50) in correspondence with these peaks, it is possible to compute an index, called α. This index consists in the square root of the ratio between the power of tachogram and systogram, corresponding to either LF or HF peaks (Cerutti et al. 1987; Robbe et al. 1987; Pagani et al. 1988b).

This approach, which requires neither preselection of data (Bertinieri et al. 1988; Legramante et al. 1999) nor injections of pressor drugs, has furnished results in man comparable (Pagani et al. 1988b) to those obtained with the phenylephrine method (Smyth et al. 1969). In addition, it enables the continuous evaluation of the minute-to-minute and circadian changes that characterize the gain of the complex baroreflex mechanisms.

Figure 30 represents an example of the results obtained with this approach. The circadian oscillation of arterial pressure, RR interval, α_{LF} and α_{HF} is well evident. In particular it is noteworthy that the α angle is remarkably similar whether obtained in correspondence of LF or HF component.

This index reached maximal values during the night and minimal ones during the day, as expected (Smyth et al. 1969), but also underwent minute-to-minute changes around its average value (Pagani et al. 1988b). This last point indicates the danger implicit in assigning one particular value for baroreflex slope in each individual in a given condition.

The index α was increased by physical training (Pagani et al.
1988b).   Conversely, it was reduced with age and during standing
(Lucini et al. 1994).

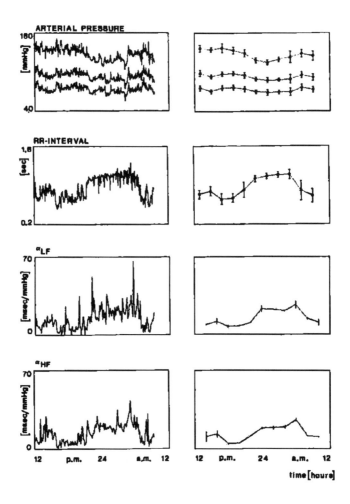

Figure 30: Arterial pressure, RR interval, αLF, and αHF, as obtained by
computer analysis of direct ECG and high fidelity intra-arterial continuous
pressure recordings during a 24-hout period. On the left panels a continuous
representation of the data. The right panels show bihourly averages with
standard deviation superimposed. (From Pagani et al. 1988b, with permission).

More elaborate models and algorithms have also been proposed in order to consider respiration together with the RR and SAP variabilities (Baselli et al. 1988). This model, by quantifying separately the effects of respiration on RR and SAP variabilities, yields the index (α) cleared of respiratory influences, and it also quantifies the effects of changes in SAP over successive SAP values.

In short, these black box approaches seem capable of evaluating the neural regulatory function and the regulated cardiovascular variables as a whole, in relation to their various functional states. The physiological mechanisms that attend this interaction need not be oversimplified.

THE INTERPRETATION OF RHYTHMS

It is remarkable to observe the conceptual differences that characterize the attempts to interpret the phenomenon of rhythmicity amongst the adepts of neuroscience, or rather of cardiovascular physiology.

As an example, Abraham et al (1973) advanced a fascinating hypothesis according to which hypothalamic electroencephalographic (EEG) waves could affect neuronal activity. The possibility of extracellular field potentials, very likely generated remotely, to influence unit activity, was conjectured as a general mechanism of brain function. Thus, more than twenty-five years ago, these authors were trying to identify the role of EEG waves in nervous function *"whether as primary information carriers or as poorly resolved epiphenomena of more basic process"*

However, in the case of cardiovascular rhythmicity, reductionistic models are in the foreground attempting to equate a rhythm to one or few reflexes, the sovereign being obviously the baroreflex (Appel et al. 1989; Eckberg 1997), discarding the possibility that rhythmicity might be a primary property carrying information.

I obviously recognize the possibility that baroreflex mechanisms might interfere with LF amplitude but always questioned (Malliani et al. 1991a) their exclusiveness in LF pattern generation. In terms of neurophysiological thinking, an increase in the rhythmicity of a neural substratum can be induced by increasing a rhythmic input to it or by reducing some tonic inhibitory activity restraining its autochthonous rhythmicity. An increased input from baroreceptors was clearly obtained by Sleight et al (1995) with their mechanical stimulation, obtained by neck chamber, but the limit of this model was, indeed, that it transformed a closed-loop system into an open input-output relation.

Usually, the tachycardia response during standing or during hypotension is attributed to a baroreflex: this attribution is obviously correct but what seems to be forgotten is that, being the baroreflex a negative-feedback mechanism, the sympathetic excitation occurs as a release phenomenon caused by a reduction of baroreceptive restraint, i.e. a reduction of the rhythmic input to the nervous centers.

Conversely, in conditions such as mental stress or physical exercise, during which there is a simultaneous presence of tachycardia and hypertension the baroreceptor firing should increase. However also in these circumstances the LF component is increased. In addition, there are conditions such as experimental myocardial ischemia during which an LF increase can occur in the absence of arterial pressure changes (Figure 28). Incidentally, in resting conscious dogs an LF component is usually present in arterial pressure variability but usually absent in RR variability, in spite of the high baroreflex gain. To further complicate this issue, the baroreflex gain is known to be decreased during standing, mental stress and exercise (Pagani et al. 1988b; Iellamo et al. 1999), conditions all characterized by an increased sympathetic activity. These are some of the reasons that convinced us to hypothesize, on pure observational grounds, that the LF rhythm seems to characterize sympathetic excitation, independently of its genesis.

In this paragraph I shall hypothesize that LF and HF correspond also to an information code, in analogy with neuroscience perspective.

Figure 31 is an adequate start for my attempt to link complexity and rhythmicity. The Figure simply indicates that LF and HF components are simultaneously present in the discharge variability of both sympathetic and vagal outputs. This Figure has been the object of a colossal misinterpretation (Eckberg 1997) trying to compare the absolute values of LF components present in sympathetic and vagal discharges. We pointed out (Malliani et al. 1998) that the comparison was not only erroneous, in view of the two different and arbitrary amplifications of the recordings, but deprived of physiological meaning.

The Figure indeed was intended to illustrate with simultaneous recordings what was already known from the literature for sympathetic and vagal activities, as summarized at the beginning of this *Chapter*.

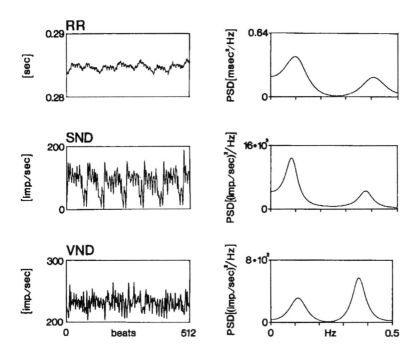

Figure 31: Spectral analysis of RR interval, preganglionic sympathetic neural discharge (SND) recorded from third left thoracic sympathetic ramus communicans, and efferent vagal neural discharge (VND) simultaneously recorded from left cervical vagus in an artificially ventilated decerebrate cat. Time series of the three signals are illustrated on left panels. A predominant LF characterizes RR and SND autospectra, whereas a greater HF component is present in VND variability. Arbitrary and different amplifications (see the ordinate scales). PSD, power spectral density. (From Malliani et al. 1991a, with permission).

However Figure 31 is also the nub of the following puzzle: if both LF and HF are present simultaneously in sympathetic and vagal discharges, how is it possible that LFnu and HFnu components of RR variability can assess the changes in sympathovagal balance? Reductionistic thinking would consider it possible only if LF component was confined to sympathetic and HF component to vagal discharge.

The view conveyed by the Figure was indeed that *"a rhythm, being a flexible and dynamic property of neural networks, should not necessarily be restricted to one specific neural pathway to carry a functional significance"* (Malliani et al. 1991a, 1998).

The core of what we propose (Malliani 1995, 1999a; Malliani et al. 1991a; Montano et al. 1998), is that two main rhythms, one marker of excitation and intrinsic in sympathetic excitation (LF) and the other marker of inhibition and quiet and linked to vagal predominance (HF), would, in physiological conditions, be organized in a reciprocal manner. The normalization procedure, in this sense, is not the result of serendipity but rather a tool to explore this hypothesis. If one accepts that cardiovascular variability generates music rather than noise (Appel et al. 1989) one should also accept that music does not rely principally on decibels (i.e., absolute power) but on notes (i.e., frequencies) and on their relationship (including relative intensity), although some power is needed for the existence of notes.

I have already expressed the opinion that both these rhythms and a large part of variance are likely to arise from a continuous interaction (Malliani et al. 1991a). Two further examples might be worthwhile. First, in the acute phases after the lesion, quadriplegic patients can have a lower than normal variance (Inoue et al. 1990; Guzzetti et al. 1994a) in the presence of an intact vagal circuitry and, often, of a resting bradycardia. Second, Introna et al (1995) have reported that in patients undergoing spinal anesthesia, when the spread of spinal block reached the highest thoracic segments (above T3), a remarkable abatement of variance and of both spectral components occurred. These observations suggest, in addition, that variance cannot be considered as a pure effect of vagal activity – as numerous authors still seem to think – but reflects a more complex interaction, although maneuvers abating vagal tone can drastically reduce variance. Thus, subtractive reasoning does not necessarily lead to bidirectional conclusions.

The study of complexity is more advisable on the basis of *what* occurs rather than *how* it may occur.

The genesis of rhythms

In the case of LF component, the hypothesis emerges more explicitly: vasomotion appears necessary at least as a sort of jogging for the vessels (to keep them in shape and ready to respond). Relatively similar rhythmic frequencies probably have to characterize the vascular smooth muscle machinery and the neural mechanisms which modulate it. In this way the vasomotor activity from a stochastic process becomes a rhythm.

On the other hand, respiration influences in a rhythmic way most of cardiovascular and respiratory afferents. It is conceivable that the neural outputs redistributed back to respiratory and cardiovascular sites maintain the same rhythmicity, again to avoid the predominance of stochastic interactions (which, still, are likely to occur).

However, two basic disturbances like vasomotion and respiration might be transformed by *the wisdom of the body* (Cannon 1932) into a code providing information to the most various central structures about the state of excitation-inhibition balance characterizing the various patterns of the organism (Malliani 1995). A similar reciprocal organization was hypothesized by Hess (1957) for the two general behaviors that he ascribed to the integration by diencephalic structures. Thus the spectral methodology could underscore the state of this balance, both at central and peripheral levels, according to a closed-loop conception.

In fact, both LF and HF components appear to be widely distributed among medullary neurons involved in the regulation of cardiovascular function (Montano et al. 1996b). It should be pointed out that these experiments were carried out in sino-aortic denervated cats, and that in some instances an LF component was present in the medullary neuron discharge variability but absent in the arterial pressure variability spectrum (Figure 32).

Thus, once again, a primary baroreceptive origin was at least unlikely. Incidentally, further demonstration ruling out the necessary role of baroreceptor mechanisms was obtained by Cooley et al (1998), who found LF oscillations in native heart RR variability of patients with left ventricular assist device and no such oscillations present in arterial pressure.

However, the most impressive finding in favor of the wide distribution of these oscillations consisted in detecting LF and HF components in the sympathetic nerve discharge, RR interval and SAP variabilities of cats after high cervical spinal section and bilateral vagotomy (Montano et al. 1996a). In these and in subsequent experiments, a transient anesthesia was administered in order to perform a midcollicular decerebration followed by suction of the forebrain, after which a bilateral cervical vagotomy and a spinal section at C1 were made, resulting in an unanesthetized spinal preparation.

It was impressive to observe (Montano et al. submitted) that in these conditions a moderate rise in arterial pressure, obtained with aortic constriction, induced a marked increase in sympathetic efferent

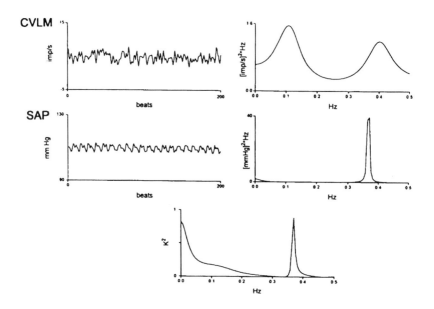

Figure 32: Spectral analysis of the discharge variability of a caudal ventrolateral medullary neuron (CVLM) and of systolic arterial (SAP) variability. The two panels on the left are the time series of the signals, while those on the right display the power spectra of their variabilities. In this case the LF and HF component are clearly evident in the CVLM spectrum, while an HF component only is present in the SAP spectrum. The bottom panel indicates the coherence (K^2) between the two signals, being significant only in correspondence of the HF component. Data are from an urethane-anesthetized cat. (From Montano et al. 1996b, with permission).

activity, through a positive feedback sympathosympathetic excitatory spinal reflex. During this reflex sympathetic excitation both LF and HF components of sympathetic discharge variability were increased in their absolute values. Interestingly, LF and HF components when expressed in normalized units were unchanged during sympathetic excitation.

Thus the reciprocal changes that most often characterize the responsiveness of LFnu and HFnu seem to depend upon a supraspinal integration as they were present in decerebrate animals (Montano et al. 1992) but undetectable during a spinal reflex. Dorsal root section from C6 to T8 vertebral segments abolished the reflex sympathetic excitation.

In short the contribution of spinal mechanisms to the genesis of LF oscillations seems demonstrated.

The presence of the HF component in RR and SAP variabilities of spinal animals is explained by the positive-pressure artificial ventilation that is capable of markedly affecting hemodynamic conditions. However, the mechanical stimulus related to ventilation was also likely to activate somatic and visceral afferents projecting to the spinal cord and thereby spinal reflex mechanisms contributing to the presence of HF component in sympathetic discharge (Sica et al. 1997). Indeed, after dorsal root section, coherence between ventilation and sympathetic spectral components was no longer present. On the other hand, HF_{RR} and HF_{SAP} oscillations have been observed also in heart transplanted patients (Bernardi et al. 1989).

Solving the puzzle

The hypothesis of a central balance between excitation and inhibition coupled with the pattern of sympathovagal balance, offers the key for solving the puzzle of the interpretation of RR variability power spectrum.

A state of excitation would be accompanied by an increased sympathetic activity with its rhythmic characteristics, conveying at the periphery the predominance of LF component; conversely, the contribution of vagal activity to the LF component would be minimal because vagal activity would be simultaneously inhibited.

On the other hand, a state of inhibition, such as that occurring during reflexes mediated by vagal afferents, would be accompanied by an increased vagal activity conveying at the periphery the increase in HF component.

In resting conditions LF and HF, both likely to have a central and peripheral mixed origin, would reflect, in their normalized values or as LF/HF ratio, the state of the central balance between excitation and inhibition coupled with the pattern of sympathovagal balance.

Thus, in spite of the redundancy of neural rhythms, they may possess the information content of a code. Some experiments can address this hypothesis. For instance, power spectral analysis of the variability of sympathetic activity recorded both in human subjects (Figure 23) and experimental animals (Figure 27), clearly indicate the importance of appreciating the different spectral profiles accompanying different states of sympathovagal balance.

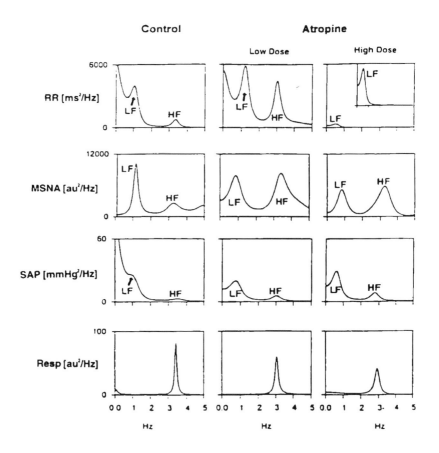

Figure 33: Spectral oscillations of RR interval, MSNA, SAP, and respiration in a normal subject during control measurements and after low-dose and high-dose atropine. After low-dose atropine (center), there is an increase in relative dominance of HF component of RR interval and MSNA. After high-dose atropine (right), RR oscillations are affected by effects of peripheral muscarinic blockade. Nevertheless, a relative increase in HF component of MSNA is evident. Because of blockade of vagal effects on heart by high-dose atropine and a decrease in RR interval variance, residual oscillatory component of RR interval is limited predominantly to LF, as seen in 15-fold magnified window. (From Montano et al. 1998, with permission).

However, in this sense, the recent experiments by Montano et al (1998) appear particularly relevant. In normal human subjects, low-dose atropine, known to exert central vagotonic effects, was found to induce bradycardia, accompanied by a decrease in LFnu and an increase in HFnu of RR variability, and a parallel decrease in LFnu and increase in HFnu of MSNA variability power spectrum (Figure 33). After high-dose atropine, in spite of muscarinic receptor blockade, the same spectral pattern was observed in MSNA variability spectrum. Thus with high-dose atropine while the sympathetic unopposed modulation consequent to muscarinic blockade was reflected, at the periphery, by the predominance of LFnu of RR variability, the vagotonic central effects of atropine could still be underscored by the predominance of HFnu in MSNA variability. Hence the detection of the two rhythms from the same neural output can in fact offer a window on the central pattern organization.

As we have recently argued (Malliani et al. 1998) the concept of sympathovagal balance coupled to the push-pull pattern of these two rhythms might have furnished the Rosetta stone that made decipherable the puzzle of the short-term oscillations imbedded in HRV.

In this perspective, however, additional notions become essential to fully appreciate the complexity of the matter. First, it has to be realized that synaptic transmission is not linear because the postsynaptic current caused by one action potential depends on the timing of the previous action potentials (Gerstner et al. 1997). Second, phenomena like synchronization are likely to serve to dynamically define neuronal populations and thereby contribute to pattern organization. Third, neural codes are not simply based on "firing rate" ("intensity code"), but rather on precise patterns (Gerstner et al. 1997) such as those describing the relationship between spectral components rather than their simple changes in absolute power. Concerning the sympathetic neural discharge, as recorded in humans and experimental animals, it is our hypothesis that the *rhythmic* code provides additional information in respect to the *intensity* code.

The exploration in the frequency domain of cardiovascular neural regulation seems to disclose a unitary vision hard to reach through the assemblage of more specific but fragmented pieces of information. Hence, a new way of thinking, seems necessary to address a territory and concepts that can only be partly quantified (Goldberger 1999), like intelligence, emotion or homeostasis (Malliani et al. 1998).

Surely, the perusal of detecting some fragments of a neural code that assumes a rhythmic vest might appear presumptuous. But science has to dare. Supposedly Albert Einstein one day said: *"I want to know God's thoughts, the rest are details"*.

Chapter 4
PATHOPHYSIOLOGICAL ALTERATIONS OF SYMPATHOVAGAL BALANCE

Tools which are more adequate to explore pathophysiology are not necessarily the most suitable ones to interpret physiology. In this *Chapter*, among other issues, the usefulness of applying both the concept of sympathovagal balance and its frequency domain assessment to the study of pathophysiological mechanisms will be analyzed. Numerous limitations will emerge, together with evident advantages. However, some initial considerations on the characteristics of a tool capable of exploring abnormalities in cardiovascular neural regulation might be appropriate.

Requirements for a tool
What is required is the capability of detecting alterations that may vary from the most drastic to only slight ones, yet crucial to interpret the ongoing pathophysiological process. Thus, it is no surprise that an adequate methodology is of paramount importance. In addition, some uncertainty is also intrinsic in the matter under scrutiny. To take an example, a continuous electrocardiographic recording from a normal subject under resting conditions, especially when analyzed with a time-frequency spectral methodology (Jasson et al. 1997; Furlan et al. 1998b), displays continuous oscillations in amplitude and frequency of spectral components: it is a common laboratory experience that sudden emotionally charged thinking during the recording is capable of markedly altering the spectral profile. Hence the sensitivity of this approach to changes that would presumably be undetectable by any other currently available technique, also represents a possible shortcoming for clinical studies.

Yet, under well controlled laboratory conditions the short and long-term reproducibility of frequency domain measurements appeared to be consistent, especially when a stimulus like head-up tilting was used in order to shift the sympathovagal balance (Pagani et al. 1986b; Pitzalis et al. 1996).

Ageing (Pagani et al. 1986b; Lipsitz et al. 1990; Montano et al. 1994) and gender differences (Huikuri et al. 1996a; Barnett et al. 1999; Fagard et al. 1999) should also be taken into careful account. Ageing, although it produces a progressive reduction of variance and hence of spectral components in absolute units, does not modify the LF/HF ratio (Pagani et al. 1986b). This suggests that a dynamic equilibrium between the modulatory influences exerted by the two branches of the autonomic nervous system exists at all ages (Fagard et al. 1999), a phenomenon that can hardly be appreciated by measuring an isolated output. Interestingly, heritable factors (Singh et al. 1999) seem to explain a substantial proportion of HRV that, therefore, should not be purely ascribed to environmental factors.

However, what has to be emphasized and has always been stressed by the promoters of this approach, is that power spectrum analysis of HRV does not provide measurements of sympathetic and vagal activities, but only markers of sympathetic and vagal modulations and of their interaction (Malliani et al. 1991a; Malik and Camm 1993; Task Force 1996). This crucial point is often forgotten by neophytes and repeatedly discovered by detractors (Eckberg 1997; Grassi and Esler 1999).

Moreover, an adequate responsiveness of cardiovascular targets, and in particular of sinus node activity, to neural modulation needs to be present in order to apply spectral methodology to the assessment of sympathovagal balance. Thus, conditions like congestive heart failure, characterized by an increased concentration of circulating catecholamines and β_1 adrenergic receptor down-regulation (Packer 1998), can only provide quite complex results, as reported subsequently. On the other hand, the disappearance of an LF component in the HRV of patients with congestive heart failure (Guzzetti et al. 1995) or after myocardial infarction (Lombardi et al. 1987) is likely to indicate a diminished responsiveness of the target organ to sympathetic modulation (Malliani et al. 1994a; Lombardi 1999) and to have an ominous prognostic value.

Obviously in research we can plan to measure only what can be measured under various conditions and, on the whole, it is likely that complementary information is provided by multifarious approaches. However in this very perspective it is difficult to accept the most recent signs of an intractable skepticism towards spectral methodology (Grassi and Esler 1999), surely not based on an adequate personal experience. In fact the former Author has never published relevant articles using this methodology, and indeed has missed recognizing that spectral analysis can extract a *frequency code* from MSNA which yields additional information and the most reproducible findings (van de Borne et al. 1997); as to the latter Author, in his main publication on HRV (Kingwell et al. 1994) he used an FFT algorithm to measure the LF component between 0.07 and 0.14 Hz, an approach (Parati et al. 1990) that unquestionably leads to an underestimation of the LF component (Fagard et al. 1998).

In their attempt to state how sympathetic activity should be assessed in humans, Grassi and Esler (1999) based their opposition to spectral methodology on Eckberg's (1997) criticisms, while disregarding our reply (Malliani et al. 1998); on some contradictory findings in the literature, largely based on technical differences; on neglecting the most probative new studies (Jasson et al. 1997; Pagani et al. 1997; Malliani et al. 1997b) supporting an opposite view; on snubbing the now widely accepted marker of sympathetic vasomotor modulation – that is the LF component of arterial pressure variability spectrum; and on the article by Kingwell et al (1994).

Comparisons among tools

In *"The wisdom of the body"* (1932) Cannon wrote: *"In clinical literature there are many references to hypothetical "vagotonic" and "sympathicotonic" states and to "autonomic imbalance". The concept underlying the use of these terms is that in normal circumstances the sympathetic and the cranial divisions of the autonomic system are acting constantly in opposition to each other and that the resultant of the conflict is an equilibrium between the two. There is evidence of such opposition in some organs but not everywhere. Where such opposition does not exist a condition of "autonomic imbalance" could not be expected".*

Reality has not changed since. It follows that considering the sympathetic regulation of cardiac function independently of vagal activity should be held as almost deprived of common sense.

Spectral methodology so far is the only approach that can estimate the sympathovagal balance in laboratory and in real life conditions.

In the above mentioned study by Kingwell et al (1994) a comparison among cardiac norepinephrine spillover, MSNA and HRV spectral analysis under various conditions was attempted. In patients with pure autonomic failure, NE spillover, MSNA and LF component of HRV were all practically abolished. In one patient with dopamine beta-hydroxylase deficiency, NE spillover and LF component of HRV were low or abolished respectively, while an increase in MSNA was present. In heart-transplanted patients, MSNA was normal, NE spillover had returned to near-normal levels after more than 2 years, while HRV total power was still markedly reduced. These findings indicate that cardiac NE spillover signals mainly the state of ventricular innervation – in this case reinnervation – rather than the modulation of sinus node activity, and that spectral methodology seems to represent the most appropriate approach to assess the state of sinus node neural modulation.

However the condition of concern was represented by cardiac failure during which NE spillover was elevated while HRV LF component was reduced in both absolute and percent units. Finally, in aged subjects compared with younger ones, NE spillover and MSNA were both elevated, while HRV LF component was decreased in absolute values (percent values were not reported). However, in this very last case, it seems wiser to hypothesize a new equilibrium between sympathetic and vagal modulations progressing with ageing (Pagani et al. 1986b; Fagard et al. 1999) rather than the occurring of an unbalanced sympathetic overactivity – this new equilibrium would take into account not only the neural discharges but the target responsiveness also revealed by spectral analysis.

In addition, it is important to point out that a static comparison (Kingwell et al. 1994) is obviously incapable of clarifying the more interesting issue of how the various approaches can assess the dynamics of neural regulation.

This type of dynamic testing was carried out, for instance, by Pagani et al (1997), while measuring MSNA, RR and SAP variability during graded changes in arterial pressure. More recently, Furlan et al (2000) have performed a similar investigation during resting conditions and head-up tilt: there was a high coherence between the LF components of MSNA, RR and SAP variabilities which all increased during tilt; moreover, the increase in LFnu of MSNA was correlated with the increase of MSNA in bursts/min.

Despite the limitations of their protocol, however, Kingwell et al (1994) correctly concluded that "*the combination of cardiac NE spillover technique and HRV will allow a more comprehensive assessment of both neuronal and postsynaptic aspects of cardiac neuroeffector response*".

In these last years, as summarized in *Chapter 3*, spectral methodology has obtained its maximal achievements, totally disregarded by Grassi and Esler (1999) who, with some lack of humor, rather conclude that "*the views of the Task Force (1996) cannot in any sense be taken to be official* ".

In research, common sense suggests the use of tools which are more appropriate to the specific needs, remembering that no tool is omnipotent. MSNA is inadequate to signal cardiac denervation or reinnervation and DβH deficiency, while HRV spectral analysis is useful in all of these cases (Fallen et al. 1988; Kingwell et al. 1994; Guzzetti et al. 1996). On the other hand, neither MSNA nor NE spillover provide information on sympathovagal balance or are very practical in ambulatory patients. Conversely, I have already alluded to the fact that even in the case of congestive heart failure the study of HRV can furnish more information than suspected by Kingwell et al (1994) and Grassi and Esler (1999).

This debate is far from being purely theoretical as, for instance, it may concern issues of relevant clinical interest such as the action of cardiovascular drugs. Indeed in the case of those rapidly lowering arterial blood pressure, this action may produce a reflex cardiac sympathetic excitation facilitating life-threatening arrhythmias (Furberg et al. 1995). In the near future it may become mandatory for the clinical application of a drug to ascertain the possible occurrence of this dangerous side-effect. On the other hand, acute intravenous administration of the angiotensin-converting-enzyme inhibitor captopril, in the conscious dog, was found to exert an important inhibitory effect on cardiac sympathetic excitatory mechanisms as well as on sympathetic vasomotor control (Rimoldi et al. 1994). In both these examples, spectral analysis of RR interval and arterial pressure variability may represent the most adequate methodology so far described for assessing the induced changes in cardiovascular neural modulation.

Finally, a comparison among tools should point out that NE cardiac spillover measurements are invasive and unlikely to be obtained in a physiological fully relaxed state. MSNA, although much less stressful, is also an invasive procedure. Thus, the totally non invasive possibilities of spectral methodology should be fully taken into account not only in view of performing large scale clinical studies but also from an ethical point of view.

Human pathophysiological studies

It is impossible and out of the scope of this book to furnish a complete survey of the amazing amount of reports that have recently applied time and frequency domain analyses of cardiovascular variability signals to the study of numerous and different pathophysiological conditions. In general, two attempts have characterized these studies. The first has been to obtain prognostic markers independent of other more traditional ones – an approach that has most often been based on the use of the simplest tools, such as those pertaining to the time domain, the results of which have been quite rewarding.

Alternatively, it has also been attempted in the course of human disease to individuate and quantify those abnormal neural mechanisms that have been extensively described in *Chapter 2* and that are capable of altering the dynamics of sympathovagal balance. This second attempt has been carried out with various and sometimes highly sophisticated algorithms and has revealed, in some instances, abnormal aspects of neural regulation probably undetectable with other approaches.

The aim of this *Chapter* is to provide some clear examples of the new information that has been gathered on several abnormal states, while considering the most relevant methodological aspects and some shortcomings implicit in an impetuously developing field.

ISCHEMIC HEART DISEASE

Prognostic indices

The first description of a negative predictive value of a reduced HRV in patients with an acute myocardial infarction comes from Wolf and coworkers (1978) when they related a diminished sinus arrhythmia to increased mortality during the early in-hospital subacute phase of the disease. These authors also noticed that a slower heart rate was usually present in patients with sinus arrhythmia, suggesting a higher vagal tone.

When applied on a large scale to normal RR intervals during 24-hour Holter recordings, a reduced SD below 50 msec was found by Kleiger and coworkers (1987) to carry a relevant prognostic value, being an independent predictor of mortality. Despite the indisputable merits of this clinical observation, substantially confirmed by Farrel et al (1991), the simple interpretation of a reduced standard deviation as consequence of a decreased vagal tone and a simultaneous sympathetic predominance (Bigger et al. 1988) might not be fully adequate. During Holter recordings numerous confounders can affect the variability signal. For instance Bernardi and coworkers (1996) have clearly shown that a large amount of RR variability and of its VLF fluctuations can depend on physical activity, an observation that implies that patients in worse conditions are also likely to be characterized by a marked reduction in mobility leading to a reduced HRV.

Commercially available algorithms have also allowed frequency domain analyses providing rather redundant information with respect to what can be simply acquired with time domain approaches. Bigger et al (1992) used an FFT algorithm to obtain a single 24-hour power spectrum (which obviously could not address the circadian rhythmicity of the spectral components) subdivided into four predetermined bands of interest. In these patients studied 2 weeks after myocardial infarction, the major finding was that the subsequent 4-year mortality was significantly correlated not only with total power but also with ultra low and very low frequency powers (both below 0.04 Hz). However, as more than 90% of power was concentrated in the frequency region below 0.04 Hz, while only about 6% was found in LF and HF bands, it is not surprising that similar prognostic information was carried by both time domain measures such as SD and by this type of frequency domain analysis.

In *Chapter 5* prognostic indices obtained with the analysis of nonlinear dynamics are also reported.

Acute myocardial infarction

To adequately study the neural mechanisms accompanying the early phases of myocardial infarction, that is when they are most likely to play a role of paramount importance (Adgey et al. 1968;

Pantridge 1978), represents a surely hard task. Apart from the difficulty of seeing the patients within the first hours, numerous factors such as pain, emotion, early administration of drugs, all interfere with the study of the underlying neural mechanisms. In a recent study we attempted (Lombardi et al. 1996c) to evaluate this issue by analyzing HRV in a group of patients in whom a 20-minute ECG recording could be obtained within a mean interval of 3 hours from the onset of symptoms related to an acute myocardial infarction. Although the mean RR interval was only slightly shorter in patients with an anterior myocardial infarction, their RR variance was significantly smaller than that of patients with an inferior localization (593 ± 121 vs. 1122 ± 191 ms^2). In both groups, however, spectral analysis of HRV indicated the prevalence of LF (respectively, 73 ± 4 and 61 ± 4 nu) over HF (13 ± 2 and 22 ± 3 nu), suggesting a shift of sympatho-vagal balance towards sympathetic predominance (Figure 34). In particular, although patients with an inferior localization presented a more variable pattern, in no cases did HF prevail. One week after the acute event, an anterior infarction was still associated with a predominant LF (68 ± 3 nu) and a reduced HF (15 ± 2 nu) – i.e., to spectral signs of sympathetic activation – but at this time a significant predominance (75 ± 3 nu) was also detectable in the LF of patients with an inferior myocardial infarction, while significant differences in RR variance were no longer present.

These data suggest that the initial vagal overactivity found by Pantridge and coworkers (1981) at the onset of inferior myocardial infarction was not any longer detectable 2-3 hours after the beginning of symptomatology – however it was probably responsible for blunting the sympathetic excitation that subsequently developed also in these patients.

Patients after myocardial infarction

Lombardi et al (1987) found that 2 weeks after myocardial infarction there was a significant increase in the LFnu and decrease in HFnu component, indicating a shift of sympatho-vagal balance towards sympathetic predominance. At this stage a tilting maneuver was incapable of further increasing the LF component.

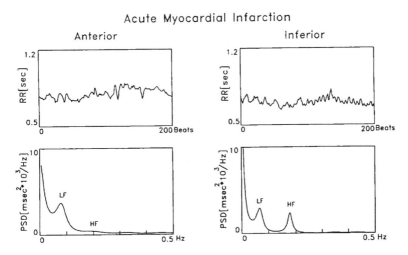

Figure 34: Spectral analysis of HRV in the acute phase of myocardial infarction. In the patient with an anterior localization (left panels) there is a clear predominance of LF, whereas in the patient with an inferior localization (right panels) LF predominates only slightly over the HF component. (From Lombardi et al. 1996a, with permission).

At 6 and 12 months a progressive decrease in the LFnu and increase in the HFnu component were observed, suggesting a normalization of sympathovagal interaction. The tilting maneuver was, in these conditions, capable again of inducing the expected increase in LFnu and decrease in HFnu component.

A sympathetic predominance and a decrease of the circadian rhythmicity of LF and HF components were observed a few days after myocardial infarction by Kamath and Fallen (1991). In a subsequent study carried out by Lombardi et al (1992), patients were studied one month after the first uncomplicated myocardial infarction, with 24-hour spectral analysis of HRV. An increased LFnu and a decreased HFnu component, as compared with control subjects were found, together with a reduction in the nocturnal increase in vagal modulation. In a similar population of patients, chronic β-blocker administration reduced the sympathetic overactivity, however without restoring a normal circadian oscillation of sympathovagal balance (Sandrone et al. 1994).

Another important aspect to be pointed out is that the spectral profile can be quite different in the presence of complicated myocardial infarction (Lombardi et al. 1996b). In Figure 35 two power spectra are presented, both obtained one month after myocardial infarction, however under quite different clinical conditions. While the patient with a normal ejection fraction presented the expected predominance of the LF component, in the patient with a reduced ejection fraction most of the energy corresponded to the VLF range. In this latter case the HF component, although markedly reduced in absolute units, but obviously prevailing in normalized units on an even smaller LF component, was likely to reflect the mechanical effects of respiration (Bernardi et al. 1989).

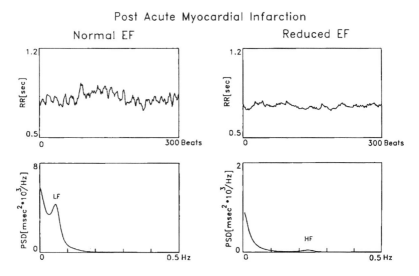

Figure 35: Spectral analysis of HRV 4 weeks after myocardial infarction in 2 patients with a normal (52%) and a reduced (28%) ejection fraction (EF). Tachograms are illustrated in the top panels. A predominant LF is evident in the autospectrum of the patient with a normal EF, whereas no LF component and a discernible HF component characterize the patient with a reduced EF. (From Lombardi et al. 1996a, with permission).

It is obvious that in these deteriorated clinical conditions, a diminished responsiveness of the sinus node to neural modulation should be taken into consideration as, among other factors, an increased concentration of circulating catecholamines and hence complex β-adrenergic receptor changes are likely to occur. However, as reported subsequently in this *Chapter* for advanced stages of congestive heart failure, the neural modulatory code is also likely to be altered.

On the other hand, it is clear that the spectral methodology should be interpreted in these conditions with relatively different criteria. For instance, in the example reported in Figure 35, it is the disappearance of an LF component of RR variability power spectrum that suggests an unfavorable clinical outcome. (Lombardi et al. 1996a; Lombardi 1999). Similar may be the interpretation of the observation by Singh and coworkers (1996) who reported that on the second day after myocardial infarction the LF/HF ratio was significantly lower in patients who died within 30 days.

However, with the frequency domain approach relevant prognostic markers have not been adequately corroborated yet.

Transient myocardial ischemia

That spectral methodology could be well suited to analyze the neural mechanisms accompanying transient myocardial ischemia was proven in conscious dogs (Rimoldi et al. 1990; Malliani et al. 1991a) in which transient occlusion of a coronary artery was accompanied by a drastic reduction in RR variance and by a marked increase in the LFnu component of HRV (Figure 28). Nonetheless, clinical studies addressing the episodes of transient myocardial ischemia occurring either spontaneously or during percutaneous transluminal coronary angioplasty have been largely inconclusive as a result of several factors. First, various transients in RR interval series are frequent; secondly, RR variance undergoes an abrupt and drastic reduction; and thirdly, ectopic beats can further complicate the picture.

In some instances, signs of clear sympathetic excitation were detectable (Malliani et al. 1994a). However, with algorithms capable of detecting transient changes, such as a time-variant analysis, the full complexity of the oscillations exhibited by neural modulation clearly emerges. Such an example is represented in Figure 36. The Figure represents a compressed array of power spectra and has to be examined from top to bottom. In the upper part of the Figure both LF and HF components can be detected in the spectral profiles. A transient ischemic episode, detected by ST-segment depression in absence of anginal pain, begins in (b) accompanied by a sudden drop of variance and practically by the disappearance of LF and HF.

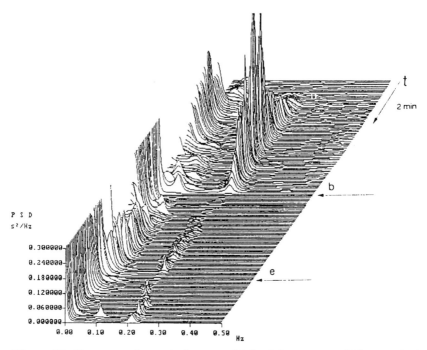

Figure 36: Compressed spectral array obtained by means of time-variant analysis of a tachogram of an ischemic episode: the beginning (b) and end (e) of the episode are marked. See text. (Modified from Bianchi et al. 1992, with permission).

However just before its beginning a prevalence of LF and a decrease of HF can be noticed. With the progression of the ischemic episode an LF component becomes again prevalent while the HF component remains depressed even after the end (e) of the episode. Marked oscillations in the VLF component also occur.

This complex spectral behavior is likely to correspond to an increased sympathetic modulation preceding the onset of transient myocardial ischemia, this shift in sympathovagal balance persisting even when ST-segment changes have vanished. However, the interpretation of the abrupt reduction in variance remains undefined as it appears too marked to be simply explained by sympathetic excitation and vagal withdrawal. An appealing hypothesis is that a sudden afferent barrage of nerve impulses coursing in both vagal and sympathetic afferent fibers (Bishop et al. 1983) might acutely disrupt central rhythmicity.

Independently of the clinical aspects of ischemic heart disease, Hayano et al (1990) studied patients undergoing coronary angiography and found in their HRV a HF component progressively decreasing with the increase in severity of angiographic abnormalities. However, the subjects were under controlled respiration and the LF/HF ratio, in all cases smaller than 1, indicated an increase in vagal modulation. Thus the results of this study can be interpreted, in my opinion, as indicating that the enhancement in vagal modulation usually induced by metronome breathing is progressively blunted in patients with angiographic coronary lesions.

On the whole, also this observation would correspond to the general principle, that has already emerged in this *Chapter*, that a reduced oscillation of the sympathovagal balance seems to represent a sensitive marker of a variety of disturbances affecting cardiovascular neural regulation.

Patients at risk of malignant arrhythmias

Despite the clinical relevance of the entire problem and the established involvement of neural mechanisms in facilitating ventricular fibrillation (Lown and Verrier 1976), little information is available on the changes in RR variability before a cardiac arrest. With a simple but ingenious analysis of heart rate fluctuations, Coumel (1990) found that an enhanced sympathetic drive was likely to precede the onset of ventricular tachycardia. On the other hand, Huikuri et al (1992) found that patients who had survived an out-of-hospital cardiac arrest were characterized by a 24-hour reduction in the average SD and HF absolute power, interpreted as reflecting a reduced parasympathetic modulation. Subsequently the same group of investigators (Huikuri et al. 1993) observed that an increase in heart rate and LF/HF ratio and a reduction in RR variance preceded the occurrence of episodes of sustained ventricular tachycardia.

Conversely, Shusterman et al (1998) observed a decrease in LF/HF before the onset of ventricular tachycardia.

Our limited experience (Malliani et al. 1994a), indicates that an increase in LFnu and LF/HF ratio is often present in the minutes preceding the onset of ventricular fibrillation (Figure 37). However, in some patients an abrupt reduction in RR variance preceding the fibrillation episode was the major finding.

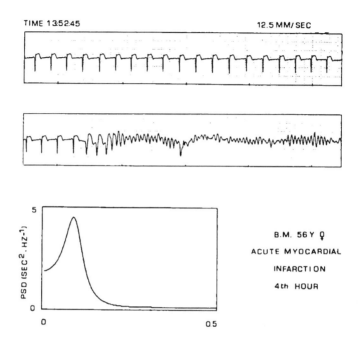

Figure 37: Spectral analysis of HRV before the onset of ventricular fibrillation (reverted with DC shock) during the acute phase of myocardial infarction. (From Malliani et al. 1994a, with permission).

In a more benign clinical setting, Wen et al (1998) also reported that a shift in sympathovagal balance towards sympathetic predominance was present from about 6 min before the onset of typical atrial flutter.

Clinical considerations

Prevention of sudden cardiac death still represents the major challenge confronting contemporary cardiology (Lown 1979). To this purpose, understanding the abnormal neural mechanisms might be of paramount importance.

From what I have summarized, it is apparent that no tool or approach seems, at the moment, capable of furnishing all the answers required. Instead, an articulated use of several criteria seems advisable.

Simple measures of HRV in the time domain are poor indicators of sympathovagal balance but, conversely, carry an important prognostic significance for patients suffering from ischemic heart disease.

However, a relevant clinical question is whether or not a sort of neurovegetative profile might characterize each individual with some predictive value about subsequent cardiac events and/or about which type of *autonomic disturbance* might be more likely to accompany such events.

However, it is in this perspective that, in my opinion, the more or less sophisticated analyses in the frequency domain can provide a quite new understanding based on the spectral profile of cardiovascular variability and on the dynamics of its neural regulation during the various laboratory and real life conditions, including the 24-hour period.

In the future, by using telemetry and adequate algorithms, it should be possible to promptly recognize the peculiarities of individual *autonomic disturbances* and to provide for them an appropriate pharmacological correction. I am convinced that this should constitute an emergency attempt paralleling the more fashionable thrombolitic procedures.

ARTERIAL HYPERTENSION

As analyzed in *Chapter 2* it is an appealing hypothesis that essential hypertension, at least in its early stages, is largely based on increased sympathetic activity. In regard to such a complex *disturbance of regulation* a veritable Pandora's box was opened by the original observation by Bristow et al (1969) that reflex lengthening in RR interval, accompanying the rises in arterial pressure induced by iv phenylephrine injection, was progressively reduced in patients with mild to more severe hypertension, as compared to normotensive subjects. These Authors correctly concluded that the described fault in cardiovascular regulation could be "*a primary disorder or secondary to the hypertensive process*".

However a large part of the subsequent research suffered from what I would consider a Ptolemaic error, in its attempt to individuate in a reduced baroreceptor restraint the cause of essential hypertension rather than a consequence of a more general abnormal disturbance leading also to hypertension.

Numerous experiments have addressed the detailed characteristics of the blunted baroreflex. However, in this fragmentation process part of the observed peculiarities was likely to depend on the experimental models. It is probably the case for the distinction according to which the reflex baroreceptor control of blood pressure would be reset but preserved, while that of the sinus node would be impaired – the residual reflex originating from carotid and not extracarotid areas (Parati et al. 1995a). However, while the carotid areas were directly stimulated with a neck chamber device, the extracarotid regions were tested by injecting phenylephrine, the widespread action of which is also capable of exciting cardiovascular sympathetic afferents. It has been amply documented in *Chapter 1* that their stimulation not only leads to sympathetic excitatory reflexes but is also capable of reducing the gain of supraspinal baroreflex mechanisms (Pagani et al. 1982; Gnecchi Ruscone et al. 1987).

It has been our long-lasting hypothesis (Malliani et al. 1975b, 1986b, 1991b) that sympathetic overactivity would depend on both an increased *"central excitatory state"* – a definition coined by Sherrington (1929) in relation to spinal integration – and a peripheral altered balance between *negative* and *positive* feedback mechanisms. In this hypothesis, the *central excitatory state* is a black box which, as an example, includes also the factors operating through the mind. The Ptolemaic error, still quite diffuse in current thinking, consists in this case in advocating, in the most disparate conditions, an altered baroreceptive function in order to explain an increased sympathetic activity and not vice versa. In my view, essential hypertension is only one of the consequences of a generalized excitatory pattern involving more variables than usually appreciated. Without denying the indisputable merits of arterial pressure measurements in the clinical and epidemiological context, it should be obvious that we measure arterial pressure also because it is very simple to do, while it is much more difficult to assess the way of thinking, the mood or the spinal excitability of a hypertensive patient.

In the conceptual approach that I propose it is essential to consider that any generalized hemodynamic stimulus activates both *negative* and *positive feedback* mechanisms and that the integrated result of a multitude of reflex circuits subserves the accompanying general pattern. Accordingly, the same stimulus produces quite different effects, depending on the various behaviors, such as wakefulness, sleep, rest, exercise (Sleight 1986; Spyer 1990). With regard to the observation by Bristow et al (1969), I hypothesize that in hypertensive patients an increased gain in the sympathetic excitatory circuits is responsible for blunting the reflex bradycardia elicitable with arterial pressure rises obtained with pressor drugs.

Given these premises, it is obvious that spectral methodology appeared to us an adequate approach to detect the possible existence of such an excitatory general pattern accompanying essential hypertension.

In an initial study (Guzzetti et al. 1988) comparing hypertensive patients with normotensive age-matched controls, it was found that in RR variability, under resting conditions, LF was greater (LF 68±3 versus 54±3 nu) and HF smaller (HF 24±3 versus 33±2 nu) in hypertensive patients. Moreover, considering the entire population of normotensive, borderline and hypertensive subjects a slight but significant positive correlation was present at rest between the LFnu component and the severity of hypertension as expressed by diastolic blood pressure levels (r = 0.30, p<0.01). This quite interesting finding, confirmed by Lucini et al (1994) and by our ongoing studies, appeared however elusive in other reports (Radaelli et al. 1994; Lazzeri et al. 1998) as it is likely to depend on numerous factors among which the stage of hypertension, the sex (Huikuri et al. 1996), the salt intake (Piccirillo et al. 1996), and previous pharmacological treatment. Hence large scale studies appear necessary to obtain a conclusive evidence.

However in the same study by Guzzetti et al (1988) it was also found that passive tilt produced smaller increases in LF in hypertensive patients than in normotensive controls (Δ LF = 6.3±2.7 versus 26.3±2.7 nu). The altered effects of tilt were also significantly correlated with the degree of the hypertensive state, suggesting a continuum distribution (r = -0.38, p<0.001).

This reduced responsiveness to tilt or to an upright position has been constantly confirmed by subsequent studies (Radaelli et al. 1994; Yo et al. 1994; Huikuri et al. 1996) and appears by now a soundly proved characteristic of essential hypertensive patients. Concerning SAP variability, Furlan et al (1991) reported an LF_{SAP} component significantly higher in hypertensive patients as compared with normotensive subjects (12±3 versus 5±1 $mmHg^2$).

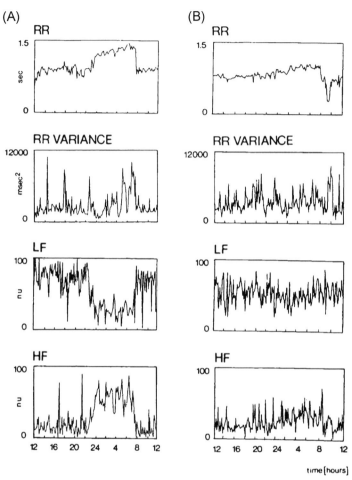

Figure 38: Comparison of the 24-hour power spectrum analysis of RR interval variability in (A) a normotensive subject and (B) a hypertensive patient. Note in (A) the marked and abrupt changes in RR interval and in LF and HF components at the moment of waking (approximately 8.00h) and the clear reduction of LF and increase of HF during the night. In (B) only a less abrupt change in RR interval occurs at the moment of waking. (From Guzzetti et al. 1991a, with permission).

However during tilt LF_{SAP} increased less in hypertensive (9 ± 6 mmHg^2) than in normotensive subjects (33 ± 8 mmHg^2). These findings were confirmed by Akselrod et al (1997) who, by using a time-variant spectral analysis, could also follow the instantaneous changes in neural modulation without observing peculiar differences between normotensive and hypertensive subjects. However, these data obtained with spectral methodology would indicate that an altered sympathetic modulation of vasomotor activity is present in hypertensive patients, which differs from the conclusions by Parati et al (1995b) using a neck chamber device.

RR variability was also studied (Guzzetti et al. 1991a) throughout the 24-hour period with Holter recordings. In the example of Figure 38 while a normotensive subject was characterized by a clear circadian rhythmicity of all represented variables, in the hypertensive patient the LFnu component did not undergo a circadian oscillation, a small nocturnal increase in HFnu being still detectable. When two groups of 30 normal subjects and 49 hypertensive patients were compared, it was confirmed that the day-night differences were marked and significant in normotensive subjects and undiscernible in the hypertensive patients (ΔLF 17±4 and 1±4 nu, p<0.01, respectively). Furthermore, the difference between daytime and night-time LFnu values was progressively reduced with increasing severity of the hypertensive state, as assessed by resting diastolic arterial pressure levels (r= -0.32, p<0.01).

A loss of circadian rhythmicity of the LF_{RR} component was also reported by Chakko et al (1993) and assessed again by Guzzetti et al (1994b).

On the other hand, in an invasive study (Pagani et al. 1988) in normotensive and hypertensive subjects undergoing 24-hour continuous recording of ECG and arterial pressure measured with a high-fidelity technique, the overall gain of the baroreceptive mechanisms was evaluated with the index α, as explained in *Chapter 3*. This index underwent a clear circadian variation, being smaller during the day (Figure 30), and was found to be decreased at rest in hypertensive as compared to the normotensive subjects (4±1 versus 10±2 msec/mmHg). Finally it was found that these peculiar changes characterizing hypertensive patients could be reversed by physical activity: indeed after a 6-month training period, LFnu of RR variability was significantly reduced and HFnu increased; moreover the index α was also significantly increased.

In a subsequent study (Lucini et al. 1994) carried out with noninvasive techniques, when the arterial pressure was continuously measured with the Finapres device, more information was obtained from a larger population of subjects. The index α was again found to be reduced, in resting conditions, in hypertensive patients as compared to controls (8±1 versus 15±2 msec/mmHg). Moreover, in both groups the index α was decreased upon standing, the reduction being smaller in hypertensive patients. The index α was also negatively correlated with age. However, the slope of the regression became flat in both groups when the subjects were examined during active standing, that is a condition of increased sympathetic modulation.

As expected, chronic β-adrenoceptor blockade, not only reduced LFnu and increased HFnu component of RR variability, but augmented the index α in both normotensive and hypertensive patients, the changes being greater in the former ones.

These findings point to the fundamental role played by the sympathetic drive in determining the gain of baroreceptor control of heart rate and its relationship with other important determinants, such as age or physical activity. Thus the reduction of baroreceptor mechanisms observed at rest in essential hypertension seems linked to the simultaneous alterations of the sympathovagal balance regulating heart period. Also in this case, however, the closed-loop relationship and the complexity of the underlying neural mechanisms discourage a simple causality interpretation (Pagani et al. 1988b).

CONGESTIVE HEART FAILURE

The abnormal neural mechanisms that accompany the evolution of the disease have already been summarized in *Chapter 2*. The study of HRV with Holter recordings has been mainly adopted in order to detect some of these mechanisms. Among the first studies, Casolo et al (1989) reported a time-domain reduction of RR variability in patients with congestive heart failure. Saul et al (1988) used instead spectral methodology and, in addition to a reduced HRV, observed that in patients with chronic congestive heart failure (class III or IV) spectral power was drastically reduced above 0.04 Hz, being mainly concentrated in the VLF region around 0.015 Hz. In these same patients heart rate also underwent very low frequency oscillations, that were often associated with a similar Cheyne-Stokes-like pattern present in respiratory activity. These Authors concluded that only sympathetic activity was being modulated significantly by this respiratory pattern, thus introducing the fundamental issue of controlling, especially in pathophysiological conditions, the respiratory activity before interpreting RR variability spectral profile. And this is indeed a precise shortcoming of studies performed with Holter recordings in which respiratory movements are not yet monitored.

A marked reduction in parasympathetic cardiac modulation in patients with congestive heart failure was reported by Binkley et al (1991) on the basis of the reduction of HF component of RR variability.

In controlled laboratory conditions, Guzzetti et al (1995) studied patients with congestive heart failure also in relation to their New York Heart Association functional class. In NYHA class II patients, hence with symptoms of mild severity, RR variability power spectrum indicated a predominance of LFnu component (Figure 39) which was however unchanged during tilt.

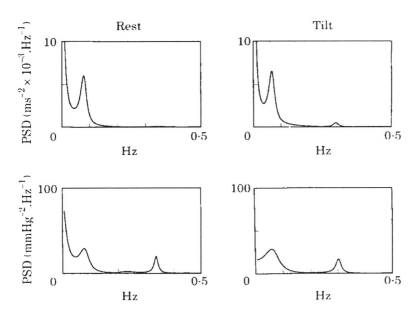

Figure 39: Spectral analysis of RR (top) and SAP (bottom) variability in an NYHA class II patient at rest and during tilting. Notice the predominance of the LF component at rest unmodified during tilting in RR variability spectra. (From Guzzetti et al. 1995, with permission).

Patients in class III presented at rest a pseudonormalization of the spectral pattern expressed in nu, but not in absolute units which were reduced as a consequence of the concomitant decrease in variance. Finally patients in class IV were characterized at rest by a very small LF component which was almost absent during tilting. In some patients in class III and IV a narrow component was noticed in the VLF region of both RR and SAP power spectra (Figure 40).

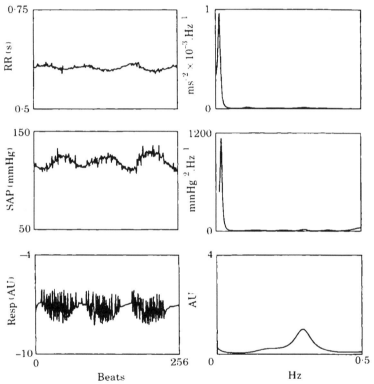

Figure 40: Example of RR, SAP and respiratory variability (left column) and corresponding spectra (right column) in a patient with a very low frequency peak at 0.018 Hz. AU = arbitrary units. (From Guzzetti et al. 1995, with permission).

It was found that this oscillatory component was correlated with the periodic changes in the amplitude of the respiratory signal (Figure 40, bottom left panel) that does not appear in the frequency domain analysis of respiration (Figure 40, bottom right panel) – to this purpose an algorithm detecting both amplitude and frequency changes would be necessary.

In most of the patients with an advanced degree of cardiac failure and a marked reduction in HRV, Mortara et al (1997) detected a discrete VLF component, accounting for a large part of total power (up to 87%), that could be ascribed to an abnormal respiratory pattern.

These findings stimulate different considerations. The shift in sympathovagal balance towards sympathetic predominance in class II patients occurred in the absence of a significant change in arterial pressure and was thus likely to be independent of baroreceptive mechanisms and largely mediated by the excitation of cardiovascular sympathetic afferents as amply discussed in *Chapter 2* – a pathophysiological aspect ignored even by the most recent review articles still proposing the initiating role of baroreceptors (Schrier and Abraham 1999). At this early stage of the disease, spectral methodology seems highly appropriate to detect this crucial sympathetic excitation. Subsequently, the progressive reduction of variance and hence of the absolute values of spectral components, paralleling the evolution of the disease, as in the case of complicated myocardial infarction, suggests an altered responsiveness of sinus node pacemaker cells (Lombardi et al. 1996a; Lombardi 1999).

However the reality turned out to be even more complex. In a recent study by van de Borne et al (1997) it was found that when an LF component was absent in RR variability it was also undetectable in MSNA variability power spectrum.

To hazard an interpretation, I would suggest that in the presence of low-pressure area congestion, the sympathetic afferent input is highly excited but without its rhythmical activity (Lombardi et al. 1976; Malliani 1982) and thus induces a reflex increase in the sympathetic efferent discharge also devoid of normal oscillations. In those same conditions of chronic sympathetic overactivity the sinus node responsiveness is likely to be reduced. Once more the closed-loop relationship would make it impossible, and somehow useless, to assess which phenomenon comes first, while instead 'it indicates quite clearly the strict connection between LF_{RR} and LF detectable from a sympathetic discharge like MSNA.

Concerning the use of time-domain analysis of HRV as a prognostic indicator (Ponikowsky et al. 1997; Nolan et al. 1998) the growing evidence is not yet conclusive. However, also in this case, it has to be considered that physical activity (Bernardi et al. 1996) and respiration can profoundly affect HRV assessed with Holter recordings.

In addition, without questioning the merits of obtaining prognostic information with a fully mechanistic approach, it would be quite interesting to compare the predictive power of the various new indexes tested in the different pathophysiological conditions with that of a thoroughly collected patient history or, better, with an elementary clinical appraisal of the remaining possibilities of performing daily physical activity.

VASOVAGAL REACTION

This pattern that often culminates in syncope is a common clinical event, the pathogenetic mechanisms of which are still poorly understood.

The term vasovagal syncope was introduced by Lewis (1932b) to signify that both blood vessels and the heart are involved. In his study there was a clear indication that the abrupt slowing of the heart rate is vagally mediated, as atropine prevented bradycardia: however the drug had little or no effect on hypotension (Lewis 1932b). Simultaneous vagal activation and sympathetic inhibition during fainting can be regarded as the hallmark of this pattern for which two different mechanisms have been hypothesized (van Lieshout et al. 1991). The first, mainly based on central neural mechanisms explains those cases in which violent emotions or severe pain lead to syncope. The second, conversely, is mainly centered upon an abnormal peripheral input originating from the heart itself.

In this regard the experiments by Öberg and Thorén (1972) had a conceptually relevant role. These Authors found that rapid hemorrhage or blood pooling, obtained with the occlusion of both caval veins, were accompanied by a reflex bradycardia often preceded by an increased impulse activity of nonmyelinated vagal afferent fibers with receptors located in the left ventricle. The same receptors were also stimulated by the obstruction of the ascending aorta and mechanical stimulation of the heart and hence had mechanoreceptive properties. Öberg and Thorén (1972) hypothesized that with rapid emptying of the heart when the unfilled ventricles contract vigorously, the receptors are excited by an improper squeezing of the myocardium, thus inducing a reflex bradycardia. In short, the main determinants of this increased impulse activity seem to be the wall deformation and an increased inotropic state of cardiac muscle.

This phenomenon seems to represent, somehow, an exception, because the vagal myelinated (Recordati et al. 1971) and the sympathetic myelinated and nonmyelinated afferents (Malliani 1982) have been found to decrease their discharge during a reduction in venous return.

On the whole, a widely accepted scheme of a typical vasovagal reaction includes a standing young subject, progressive sympathetic excitation and reduction of venous return, until a switch becomes operative and a sudden excitation of vagal and inhibition of sympathetic outflow occur.

Figure 41 represents a typical case of syncope during a tilt test, analyzed with spectral methodology.

In 1, during rest, both LF and HF components are detectable in the RR variability spectrum, while during tilt only an LF component is practically present. During this state of marked sympathetic overactivity the syncope occurs suddenly.

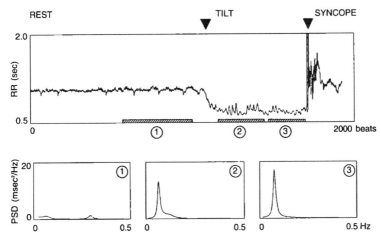

Figure 41: RR variability spectrum of an apparently normal subject, 18y, at rest (1) and during tilt at 90°. The early asympatomatic phase corresponds to (2), while the period closer to syncope corresponds to (3). Upper panel reports the continuous tachogram. (From Furlan et al., unpublished observations).

However, when the changes in neural modulation were analyzed with algorithms capable of assessing the time development of frequency components, thus providing information in both time and frequency domain, the pattern appeared less uniform. In a study by Furlan et al (1998b), using a time-variant autoregressive approach, two different time courses of spectral changes were present in 22 healthy subjects who experienced fainting for the first time during a 90° head-up tilt.

Figure 42 presents (left panels) the usual findings during tilt in a control subject, characterized by stable RR interval, sustained increase in LFnu and decrease in HFnu, despite some oscillations.

The two autonomic patterns leading to fainting have been indicated as *sudden syncope* (middle panels) and *syncope with latency* (right panels).

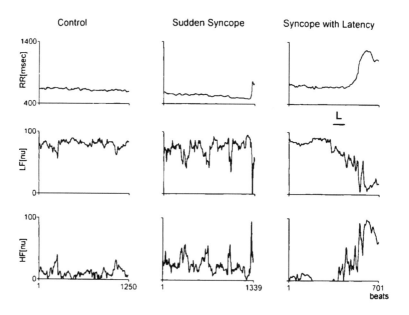

Figure 42: Tilt procedure in a control (left) and in two subjects who suffered from syncope (center and right). Latency (L) is arbitrarily defined as time lag between maximum reached by LFnu component during tilt and onset of bradycardia. (From Furlan et al. 1998b, with permission).

The subject with *sudden syncope* had a slight decrease of RR and a progressive increase of LFnu, paralleled by a reduction of HFnu until syncope occurred, accompanied by sudden rise of RR and HFnu and drop of LFnu. Of interest, LFnu exhibited large fluctuations during the entire tilt period. In the case of *syncope with latency* LFnu component, after an initial plateau, underwent a slow decrease, with a final reduction at the time of syncope. In addition, a marked progressive increase in HFnu was evident during the period preceding the maximal bradycardia. Consequently, a latency between the maximal level reached by LFnu and the onset of bradycardia could be identified.

Of the 22 subjects who developed syncope, 13 suffered from a *sudden syncope*, while the 9 remaining patients were characterized by a time lag between the maximum of LFnu and the onset of bradycardia (range from 12 to 167 seconds).

It is clear that the spectral findings accompanying *sudden syncope* lend further support to the original hypothesis by Öberg and Thorén (1972), in which a marked sympathetic excitation plays a major role. Conversely, the pattern characterized by a progressive sympathetic inhibition suggests that additional pathophysiological mechanisms are likely to interact. In this perspective, Morillo et al (1994) found reduced values of LF and LF/HF during the first 5 minutes of a 60° tilt, suggestive of a failure in vagal withdrawal and a blunted sympathetic activation (Dickinson 1993). Similarly, Lepicovska et al (1992), using a time-frequency mapping of RR variability, concluded that subjects prone to vasodepressor syncope were characterized by an elevated cardiac parasympathetic activity that persisted during orthostatic stress.

The two patterns represented in Figure 42 are close to the extremes of the observed divergence and therefore it is likely that a relevant overlap of mechanisms occurs in most cases of fainting. However this dichotomy, revealed by a more sophisticated spectral methodology, not only further emphasizes the complexity of these patterns but suggests that different therapies may be indicated in the prevention of syncopal events, ranging from β-adrenergic receptor antagonists to α-adrenergic receptor agonists.

ORTHOSTATIC HYPOTENSION AND INTOLERANCE

Pure autonomic failure

This rare neural degenerative condition is characterized, during the assumption of orthostatic posture, by a relevant decrease in systemic arterial pressure which is not attended by any compensatory change in heart rate (Bradbury and Egglestone 1925).

A defect in the sympathetic branch of the autonomic nervous system seems to be its main feature, as indicated by pathological and pharmacological studies. In fact, catecolamine fluorescence, assessed by means of histochemical techniques, is defective in perivascular sympathetic endings examined with muscle biopsy, indicating a reduction in available norepinephrine (Kontos et al. 1975).

Moreover, in patients affected by pure autonomic failure, indirect evidence of an alteration of the sympathetic nervous system is also provided by the lack of a vasoconstrictor response to intra-arterial tyramine (Kontos et al. 1975; Bannister 1979), which is an indirectly acting amine promoting norepinephrine release from sympathetic nerve endings. Accordingly, in these patients, intra-arterial norepinephrine produced an enhanced vasoconstriction as usually observed in denervated tissues (Kontos et al. 1975; Bannister 1979). Finally, as already mentioned, cardiac NE spillover and MSNA were found to be almost abolished in this condition (Kingwell et al. 1994).

On the other hand, although · no direct evidence of morphological alterations involving the vagal nerves has yet been provided by pathological studies, a dysfunction in the parasympathetic cardiac control was already hypothesized many years ago by Bradbury and Egglestone (1925) on the basis of the finding that an increase in arterial pressure induced by epinephrine or the head-down posture did not induce a bradycardia response. Moreover, Ibrahim et al (1974) observed a lack of change in heart rate after atropine administration.

Spectral methodology appeared as an adequate and simple technique to simultaneously assess the state of sympathetic and vagal modulation of heart period.

Kingwell et al (1994) first reported the absence of a spectral component around 0.1 Hz in RR variability of patients with pure autonomic failure in resting conditions: however, probably due to the employed spectral methodology, the HF component as well was undetectable in HRV.

Furlan et al (1995) carried out a more detailed analysis.

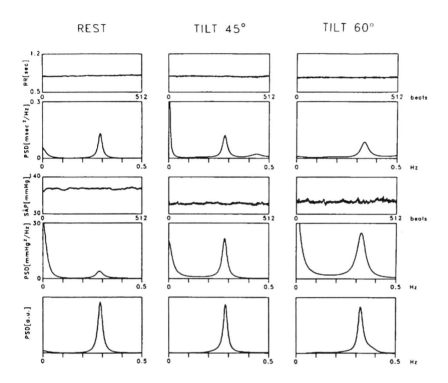

Figure 43: Example of spectral analysis of RR interval and SAP variabilities and of respiration in a patient with pure autonomic failure at rest and during 45° and 60° head-up tilt. Notice that, at rest as well as during the sympathetic stimuli (45° and 60° tilt), the only detectable oscillatory component in RR interval and SAP variabilities is the high frequency oscillation (HF), synchronous with respiration. Power spectral ordinates for RR variability should be multiplied by 10^3. (From Furlan et al. 1995, with permission).

In 4 patients with pure autonomic failure, RR interval variance was found extremely reduced with respect to control subjects, while SAP variance was not so drastically diminished. Moreover, as exemplified in Figure 43, an LF component was absent in RR and SAP variability spectra, both at rest and during graded tilt. On the other hand, the HF component was likely to simply reflect the mechanical effects of respiration (Bernardi et al. 1989) as its absolute power was not significantly modified by atropine administration. The baroreceptor mechanisms were evaluated with the index α (Pagani et al. 1988b), calculated in correspondence of the HF components of RR and SAP variability, and appeared drastically reduced. Accordingly, phenylephrine i.v. injection produced no reflex bradycardia.

Thus the application of spectral methodology to this rare disease has furnished the expected results in regard to sympathetic modulation and has reinforced the view that in the presence of profound anatomical damage leading almost to an absence of sympathetic control, a reduction of vagal modulation may be necessary to avoid the devastating effects of an unopposed vagal predominance.

Other pathophysiological conditions, all leading to orthostatic hypotension or intolerance can be profitably explored with spectral techniques especially to determine the crucial interaction between sympathetic and vagal mechanisms. The list includes a similar but less rare condition, associated with central nervous system alterations (Blaber et al. 1996) and hence with a more severe prognosis, known as multiple system atrophy or Shy-Drager syndrome (Consensus Committee 1996). And includes also a quite frequent and usually benign, although at times invalidating, disturbance that has been labeled with various terms such as postural orthostatic tachycardia (Low et al. 1995), idiopathic hypovolemia (Fouad et al. 1986), hyperadrenergic orthostatic hypotension (Streeten 1990) and, more recently, chronic orthostatic intolerance (Furlan et al. 1998a; Narkiewicz and Somers 1998).

Chronic orthostatic intolerance

This disturbance has been estimated to affect more than 500,000 people in the United States, its prevalence being higher in young women (female to male ratio 4:1). Symptomatology is characterized by an exaggerated tachycardia without hypotension and by signs of orthostatic intolerance such as fatigue, lightheadedness, dizziness and syncope during up-right position, although rarely. If not correctly diagnosed, the chronic inability to stand may trigger a vicious cycle leading to a remarkable reduction in physical activity which in turn aggregates intolerance to gravity.

In a recent study Furlan et al (1998a) assessed the autonomic profile of a group of patients with chronic orthostatic intolerance while recumbent and during a 75° tilt test, by using direct recording of MSNA, plasma catecholamine detection and spectral methodology applied to both RR interval and SAP variability.

In recumbent position MSNA (bursts/min) was higher in subjects with orthostatic intolerance than in controls. In addition, HR, LF_{RR}/HF_{RR} ratio and LF_{SAP} were higher in patients suggesting an enhanced cardiac and vascular sympathetic modulation compared to healthy subjects.

During the gravitational stimulus (tilt) a blunted increase in MSNA was attended by a remarkable enhancement of HR and LF_{RR}/HF_{RR} ratio. Conversely, the increase in LF_{SAP} was comparable to that present in control subjects.

This is a clear example in which the simultaneous use of different techniques has made it possible to detect a differential distribution of increased sympathetic modulation which, in upright position, seems to be directed mainly to the heart.

DIABETIC NEUROPATHY

Neuropathy is a frequent complication of diabetes mellitus, with reported frequencies ranging from 5 to 60%. The involvement of the autonomic nervous system is often suggested by symptoms like postural hypotension, impotence in the male, bladder and bowel dysfunction. However, the involvement of cardiac innervation is less easy to recognize, although eventually some patients develop a fast and fixed heart rate, as an expression of functional denervation (Lloyd-Mostyn and Watkins, 1976). The mortality of patients with autonomic dysfunction is increased dramatically (Ewing et al. 1976).

In order to recognize the early changes in cardiovascular neural control mechanisms before the appearance of clinical symptoms, a battery of 5 simple, non-invasive cardiovascular reflex tests is usually employed (Ewing et al. 1985). However, since a single test may not distinguish the severity of autonomic damage, a scoring system has been suggested. In spite of the clinical convenience of considering changes in heart rate and in arterial blood pressure as depending, respectively, upon vagal and sympathetic activities, the scoring system respects the well recognized notion that both arms of the autonomic nervous system take some part in all 5 tests (Ewing et al. 1985). In this approach, however, the need of the active collaboration of the patients in order to elicit phasic changes in heart rate and arterial blood pressure can affect the accuracy and reproducibility of the results.

Thus, also in this case, spectral methodology appeared to be a quite useful tool.

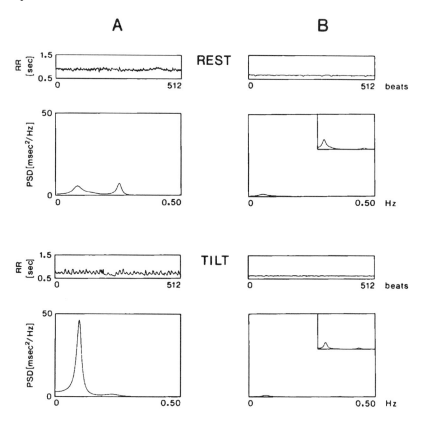

Figure 44: Representative example of RR variability in a diabetic patient with no signs of autonomic neuropathy (left panels, A) and in a patient with signs of neuropathy (right panels, B). Notice the increase in the low frequency component with tilt only in the patient without neuropathy. The two spectra of the patient with neuropathy are characterized by a very low power, i.e. small total area. Consequently, they are also shown in the insert with x10 magnification of the vertical axis. (From Pagani et al. 1988a, with permission).

Pagani et al (1988a) studied a group of 49 diabetic patients free of gross clinical signs of autonomic dysfunction and the information provided by spectral methodology was compared with that obtained from the tests score.

A significantly reduced RR interval variance, as already reported by Kitney et al (1982) and by Lishner et al (1987), was found for the whole group of patients, as compared with that of control subjects.

In patients without signs of diabetic neuropathy, as assessed by the tests score, spectral profile at rest and during tilt was not altered (Figure 44, left panels).

Conversely, in patients with signs of diabetic neuropathy assessed with the tests score, the spectral components were barely detectable and unchanged during tilt (Figure 44, right panels).

To verify the applicability of spectral analysis of RR variability to the assessment of the degree of visceral neuropathy in diabetes, a matrix of correlation was used in which spectral indices of sympathetic and parasympathetic modulation were correlated with the 5 tests score. For each test, normal response was graded 0, borderline response 0.5 and abnormal response 1, so that each patient could obtain a score 0-5, indicative of the severity of neural visceral impairment (Ewing et al. 1985).

At rest, in diabetics as in controls, RR variance was greater in younger subjects. In the group studied a significant inverse correlation was observed between RR variance and both age and tests score. However, when age and score were introduced simultaneously in the same model, score lost significance, thus indicating an important effect of age on score determinations.

As to the changes induced by tilt, those in variance were correlated with age but not with score. On the contrary, score showed a significant correlation with the changes in spectral indices induced by tilt which were larger in those patients which had a lower score. In particular, there was a weak inverse correlation between score and increase in LFnu and LF/HF, while this weak correlation assumed a positive sign when score was compared to the decrease of the HFnu reduction. Furthermore in 5 out of 6 patients that showed an opposite change in LFnu or HFnu with tilt as compared to controls, i.e. a decrease in LFnu or an increase in HFnu (Figure 45) the score was greater than 3.

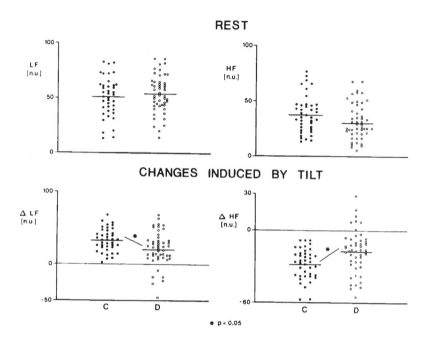

Figure 45: Comparison of spectral components of diabetics (D) and controls (C) at rest (top panels) and comparison of the changes induced by tilt (bottom panels). Notice significantly greater changes in controls. (From Pagani et al. 1988a, with permission).

With regard to a reduced oscillation of sympathovagal balance, Bernardi et al (1992) reported that also the circadian oscillation of spectral profile is markedly reduced in diabetic patients. These data, on the whole, challenge the traditional concept of an early alteration of parasympathetic modulation as a peculiar aspect of diabetic neuropathy, since the blunted oscillation of sympathovagal balance cannot be ascribed to one single component only (Pagani et al. 1988a; Bellavere et al. 1992).

Moreover, and much more importantly, in view of the clinical relevance of assessing in its early stages the existence of an autonomic neuropathy and subsequently its evolution and, hopefully, in order to individuate some therapeutical intervention, it may be important to widely promote the use of spectral methodology, as consistent findings seem to indicate it as a reliable tool in this area of clinical medicine.

CARDIAC TRANSPLANTATION

The condition after human heart transplantation represents a clinical model of denervated heart that has prompted various studies with spectral analysis (Fallen et al. 1988; Bernardi et al. 1989; Sands et al. 1989). In general, reduced total RR variance was found. However, although in some studies (Fallen et al. 1988; Sands et al. 1989) no discrete HF or LF components were consistently found in RR variability, Bernardi et al (1989) described a small HF component interpreted to be independent of neural mechanisms. Furthermore, in one patient studied 33 months after transplantation by Fallen et al (1988), both LF and HF components were present, the latter increased by synchronous respiration and abolished by atropine. It was concluded that spectral analysis could offer a unique method for establishing the state of possible reinnervation of human transplanted heart. The existence of both sympathetic and parasympathetic reinnervation was confirmed by Bernardi et al (1998), and its entity was also related to the type of surgical procedure. Indeed, when a new technique was used, involving a more extensive atrial resection and total cardiac denervation, both autonomic branches appeared to have an increased tendency to regenerate.

Finally, Sands et al (1988) reported an increased variance in patients developing an allograft rejection, a finding, that has been confirmed experimentally with rat cardiac allografts (Wada et al. 1999).

MISCELLANEA

The progressive application of the frequency domain analysis of cardiovascular signal variability to the most different areas of human pathophysiology has to mentioned.

Duchenne-type muscular dystrophy has been studied by Yotsukura et al (1988) and a shift of sympathovagal balance towards a sympathetic predominance was found.

Familial dysautonomia was investigated by Maayan et al (1987) and an altered responsiveness of sympathovagal balance was evidenced.

Neurovascular compression associated to arterial hypertension was reported by Makino et al (1999) to be accompanied by signs of sympathetic overactivity.

In *Chapter 3* some studies on subjects with complete quadriplegia (Inoue et al. 1990, 1991; Guzzetti et al. 1994a; Koh et al. 1994) have already been analyzed for their contribution to the interpretation of spectral components. Grimm et al (1997) have studied subjects with different types of spinal cord injuries and have suggested that some balance between the two autonomic components is reestablished after one component has been severely damaged.

A sympathovagal balance shifted towards vagal predominance has been described by Garrard et al (1992) in patients with bronchial asthma, while Pagani et al (1996) found a reduced responsiveness of the balance during tilt in patients with chronic obstructive pulmonary disease.

Obstructive sleep apnea was studied by Narkiewicz et al (1998) who also recorded MSNA: progression of apnea severity was positively correlated with increase in SAP variability and LFnu of RR variability.

Hypertrophic cardiomyopathy was studied by Ajiki et al (1993) and also in this case a shift of sympathovagal balance towards a sympathetic predominance was reported.

Dalla Vecchia et al (1998) studied 19 patients with a large ventricular aneurysm before and after a surgical reconstruction of left ventricular geometry accompanied by coronary artery bypass graft: while tilt test, before surgery, did not induce significant changes in spectral profile of RR and SAP variability, a clear sympathovagal balance responsiveness was restored after surgery. Similarly, Bonaduce et al (1994) reported that successful coronary angioplasty can enhance an abnormally depressed HRV.

In patients with positive serology for Chagas' disease and electrocardiographic alterations but without heart failure, RR variance and power spectral profile at rest were not different from those of control subjects; however, when patients were standing, the usual increase in LFnu and decrease of HFnu of RR variability were not present (Guzzetti et al. 1991b).

These are only a few examples. On the other hand, conditions less definable as pathological have been also studied. A sympathetic predominance was observed in obese subjects by Karason et al (1999), reversed by drastic weight loss. Similarly, a sympathetic predominance and a reduced sympathovagal responsiveness was found by Pagani et al (1994) in subjects complaining of unexplained fatigue.

Adaptive changes have also been investigated, as in the case of the study by Bernardi et al (1997) carried out on endurance runners before and after 46 Km of rocky trail at 2500 m. Prolonged exertion was associated to an increased sympathetic modulation, while long-lasting effects on cardiovascular autonomic modulation were still detectable after 24 hours.

Similarly, Furlan et al (1993) had previously reported that signs of an increased sympathetic modulation were still present in young subjects 24 hours after maximal dynamic exercise.

In the near future space flight may furnish an appropriate model to study some extreme adaptations of sympathovagal balance.

CONCLUSIONS

There can be few doubts that the application of the frequency domain analysis to the study of physiology and pathophysiology has already provided new and useful information. In addition it corresponds, in a fully reductionistic era, to the opposite need of approaching the indetermination of complex patterns. In the case of this book, this underlines the concept that disease is an innervated entity.

Combining reductionistic findings with pattern organization is surely one of the nodal points in future development. Dangers are always the same. To shrink too many findings into a concept; not to perceive the contradictions; not to realize that opposite principles can participate in the same design.

Biology does not follow an Aristotelian logic: fortunately, as it would be quite boring. Discoveries are more likely to result from sound observations than from *a priori* reasoning. The Hegelian dialectic process in which a contradiction between thesis and antithesis is resolved by synthesis at a higher level of knowledge, still appears as a valid metaphor of biological organization and of our attempt to understanding it.

The frequency code is probably a powerful key to decipher some physiological patterns and their alterations. But it requires, when used as a tool, a dialectic mind. A rhythm is a functional and dynamic property that cannot be equated to one particular reflex, as already amply discussed in this book, or to a unique state. For instance, a fully atropinized cat can exhibit an electroencephalographic rhythmicity simulating placid sleep, and yet be walking around. Nevertheless it is difficult to deny that EEG contains important information.

The so heavily disputed normalization procedure for assessing the power of LF and HF spectral components of RR variability is a tool that has provided, like the LF/HF ratio, unprecedented assessments of the changes in cardiovascular neural modulation. Any investigator is free to discard them and to find better tools, however without assuming that the frequency code contains no information.

As an example of the contradictory nature of biological findings, it is remarkable that the normalized value of LF component of RR variability, which – when increased – is a reliable marker of sympathetic excitation, is drastically reduced together with RR variance and LF absolute units in pathophysiological conditions accompanied by massive sympathetic overactivity. This is likely to be partly due to a decreased responsiveness of sinus node pacemaker cells largely depending on β-adrenergic receptor down-regulation, as a result of extremely high sympathetic discharge and circulating levels of catecholamines. Hence, in these cases, it is the progressive reduction of an LF component that signals a massive sympathetic excitation, usually associated to poor prognosis.

However, similar dynamic properties characterize also the HF component which, on the basis of its claimed pure vagal nature, is much more accepted by simplistic reasoning as a totally reliable marker of vagal modulation. Also in this case, however, to take just an interesting example, it has been reported that phenylephrine administration, clearly increasing vagal activity as reflected by simultaneous bradycardia, can abolish respiratory sinus arrhythmia (Parati et al. 1995b).

A leitmotiv of this book is the interaction of opposite mechanisms. By now we should know that in science it is inevitable to falsify and supersede established theories, according to Karl Popper's rule. However, sometimes, a more adventurous trajectory may even be preferable. Feyerabend (1975) stated that violations are necessary for scientific progress, that prejudices are identified by contrast and not by analysis, and, together with Bertolt Brecht, that science is mainly an anarchic venture.

I have often advised young investigators asking for an experimental problem to be studied, to select one area in which everything appeared established and totally explained by one single mechanism and to look for the opposite.

This *Chapter* concludes this search for an interaction of opposite mechanisms in physiology and pathophysiology. However, after *Chapter 5* that is just an additional window on a world of complexity, in *Chapter 6*, dealing with ethics, additional reasons are given to search for the opposite in science. One reason being that science is not neutral, and scientific power is often polarized.

Chapter 5
VARIABILITY AND NONLINEAR DYNAMICS

Cardiovascular signal variability and in particular HRV are only in part the result of complex rhythmical oscillations, largely corresponding to linear dynamics. Thus, several studies (Goldberger and West 1987; Guzzetti et al. 1996; Sugihara et al. 1996) have provided evidence that nonlinear dynamics is present in HRV. In fact, the system seems to display a behavior ranging from a regular periodicity to an erratic pattern which, from the geometrical and dynamical point of view, might have a deterministic rather than a stochastic nature. Hence what may be often interpreted as a noise effect could be hypothesized to pertain to a nonlinear deterministic system, extremely sensitive to initial conditions, a pattern generally assumed as defining a chaotic system (Denton et al. 1990; Glass and Mackey 1998).

The sinus rhythm system consists in the sinoatrial node activity controlled by multiple and complex neural mechanisms which constitute a near-perfect theoretical substrate for the generation of chaos (Denton et al. 1990).

The initial approaches to this problem have been mainly based on the reconstruction of the trajectory of a system evolution in the phase space. To this purpose it would be necessary to take into account a large number of physiological variables. On the contrary, a few mathematical theorems suggest that a chaotic process might be studied by looking at the realization of a time series, sufficiently long and adequately sampled, providing the invariant information that quantifies the chaotic dynamics of the system (Takens 1981). Consequently, it would be possible to draw quantitative inferences about the dynamical structure of the entire system from the behavior of a single variable.

Frequently used indexes of nonlinear dynamics include:

-   D_2 *(correlation dimension)* that estimates the number of independent variables describing the system dynamics; in the case of chaotic dynamics this number is not an integer (Grassberger and Procaccia 1983).
-   K_2 *(Kolmogorov entropy)* that estimates the amount of new information furnished by the system evolution; in the case of periodic dynamics $K_2 = 0$, while $K_2 \neq 0$ in the case of both stochastic and deterministic evolutions.
-   *H (self-similarity exponent)* that estimates the degree of geometrical fractality, indicating when the signal is self-similar while varying the temporal scale (Denton et al. 1990). $1/H$ is considered an estimation of fractal dimension.
-   *Lyapunov exponents* that measure the exponential evolution of nearby trajectories in the phase space (Eckmann et al. 1986). The exponents are negative in the case of converging trajectories, positive in the case of diverging trajectories, equal to zero in the case of periodic dynamics.

As an example, these indexes were used to compare the nonlinear dynamics present in the HRV of normal subjects and heart-transplanted patients (Guzzetti et al. 1996). D_2, K_2 and $1/H$ were significantly reduced in transplanted patients compared with controls, indicating a loss of complexity characterizing the HRV of a transplanted heart. Similarly Lyapunov exponents were significantly less positive in transplanted patients. Their positivity is often accepted as suggestive of chaotic dynamics (Eckmann et al. 1986), although stochastic time series also have a positive Lyapunov exponent. It was suggested (Guzzetti et al. 1996) that the loss of complexity which characterizes the transplanted patients might mainly depend on the interruption of neural connections between the heart and the central nervous system. However, it was noteworthy that HRV possessed characteristics of nonlinear complex behavior, also when recorded from a transplanted heart.

A significantly reduced D_2 was also found after myocardial infarction in HRV of patients with a low ejection fraction as compared with patients with a normal ejection fraction (Lombardi et al. 1996b).

These two examples allow some general considerations on the actual limits of this approach.

In general, the assessment of nonlinear dynamics, like spectral methodology, would require stationary conditions and long series of uninterrupted data (at least 10-20.000). Such time series are usually obtained with Holter recordings and hence it is obvious that the first theoretical prerequisite is not fulfilled. Even more importantly, long time series represent an almost insurmountable obstacle against the possibility of carrying out experiments with acute interventions.

The attempt to overcome this problem by oversampling the recordings and by using shorter time series (e.g. 5000 data points) does not appear as being a sound approach. However with this procedure Kagiyama et al (1999) have recently reported a reduced D_2 in HRV of hypertensive patients, compared with normotensive controls.

By now, an additional widely used index of nonlinear dynamics is known as α and corresponds to the exponent of the *1/f power law* (Kobayashi and Musha 1982). These Authors found that over a frequency range of 0.0001 to 0.02 Hz (corresponding to VLF), the relationship between the log of power and the log of frequency was described by a straight line with a slope (α) around −1, indicating that the power decreased approximately as the reciprocal of frequency (*1/f*). The index α, as a measure of fractality, corresponds to an additional estimate of *H*.

In the example of Figure 46 the slope (α) was assessed in two patients after myocardial infarction. The slope was reduced in a patient with a reduced ejection fraction (EF) (bottom) as compared with a patient with a normal EF (top). An inverse significant correlation between α and EF was found (Lombardi et al. 1996b).

Moreover, this index has proven to be an excellent predictor of all-cause mortality or arrhythmic death in patients with recent acute myocardial infarction and with heart transplant (Bigger et al. 1996).

Hence, while the application of these nonlinear dynamics indexes to the complexity of biological events seems to have a rather scarce heuristic value for the analysis of the underlying mechanisms, it might conversely offer important prognostic tools.

An additional perspective of great interest corresponds to individuating biological models which might exhibit a behavior pertaining to chaotic dynamics (Mansier et al. 1996a; Persson and Wagner 1996; Wagner and Persson 1998). Accordingly, a strategy based on the change of a control parameter in the experimental protocol and on the classification of the evoked nonlinear dynamics can be followed. This approach allows to construct a *bifurcation* diagram indicating the parameter value determining a change in the behavior of the experimental preparation. If a standard *route* is

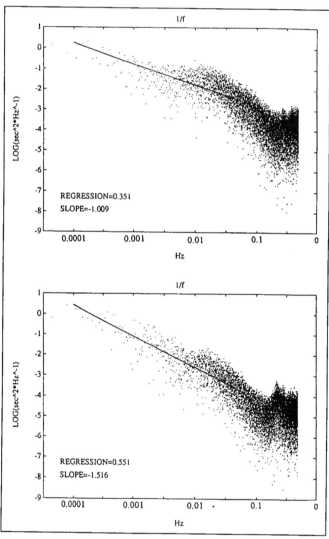

Figure 46: Log-log plot of power density and frequency of 2 patients with normal (top) and reduced (bottom) EF. The solid line represents the regression calculated in the frequency range between 0.0001 and 0.04 Hz. (From Lombardi et al. 1996b, with permission).

found, such as a period doubling cascade (Griffith 1996), the claim for chaos is more robust. This approach appears closer to physiology than a mere application of signal processing methods and can be performed over short data sequences (classification methods do not imply the use of large amount of samples).

Similarly, Guevara et al (1988) classified the nonlinear interactions between periodic trains of current pulses and the spontaneous rhythmical activity of aggregates of chick ventricular heart cells when the stimulation frequency was changed. In this way they were able to observe a period doubling *route to chaos*.

The identification of appropriate biological models of nonlinear dynamics will occupy the foreground of the following pages, and the search for adequate mathematical tools will be rather a consequence, thus inverting, somehow, the perspective presented in the initial part of this *Chapter*.

This strategy might be defined as *pattern recognition*.

Definition of nonlinear dynamics

In biology, the possibility exists of innumerable mechanisms producing nonlinear relationships (e.g. sigmoidal, exponential or logarithmic functions), all generating nonlinear dynamics and thus preventing its simple definition. Conversely, a process can be defined as linear when its properties can be completely described by a given number of oscillations with random phases. Such a linear process is totally described in the time domain by the autocorrelation function, and by the power spectrum in the frequency domain. The dynamics which do not fulfill this definition can be considered as nonlinear.

These premises should suffice to infer that the vast majority of biological phenomena has a nonlinear nature. When a flexor and an extensor muscle participate in the movement of a joint they generate a nonlinear interaction, even if their integrated action can result in a linear movement: in fact the contribution of either muscle has nonlinear characteristics as it determines only unidirectional and not bidirectional changes. When an inhibitory reflex opposes an excitatory one it is also a nonlinear interaction. In short it would appear that the entire biological scenario might be ascribed to nonlinear properties. Instead, as it has been amply analyzed in *Chapter 3*, linear dynamics has emerged in biology: and that present in HRV is likely to reflect an aspect of the mastership of neural integration.

From an investigator's point of view, an essential issue is represented by the tools to be used in order to acquire the information pertaining to the linear and nonlinear features of the same complex dynamics.

In the example of Figure 47, two simulated continuous time series with identical mean and variance are represented in the left panels (*a* and *b*). The tracing *a* swings between oscillations occurring at positive and negative values, such a switch indicating a chaotic dynamics. Simultaneously the same tracing exhibits clear rhythmical oscillations that are described by their power spectrum in *c*. The tracing *b* is the result of phase randomization (Theiler et al. 1992) of tracing *a,* leaving unchanged the rhythmical oscillations and hence their power spectrum (*d*). However the tracing *b* has lost the chaotic behavior, i.e. its swinging between two prevalent levels.

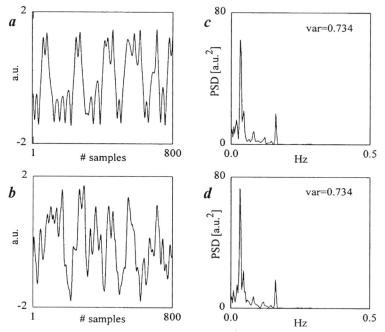

Figure 47: (*a*) tracing obtained with Duffin oscillator forced by a periodical input; (*b*) tracing obtained after phase randomization; (*c* and *d*) respective FFT power spectra. a.u.: arbitrary units; var: variance. See text. (From Porta et al.1995, unpublished observations).

This simulated example indicates that linear and nonlinear features can coexist and that it is possible to eliminate the nonlinear components with a phase randomization procedure.

Experimental studies

Figure 48 provides an example of a nonlinear phenomenon detected in the course of a physiological experiment. As already summarized in *Chapter 1*, in our search for a cardiocardiac sympathosympathetic reflex (Malliani et al. 1969), we used to record the action potentials of one single or of a few preganglionic efferent sympathetic fibers isolated from the third ramus communicans. In the panel B the upper tracing is a cathode-ray display of impulse activity: the action potentials of two fibers were simultaneously recorded, one with a predominantly negative potential (upward deflection) and one with a predominantly positive potential (downward deflection). The upward impulses were used to trigger upward pulses on a polygraph recording (B, middle tracing): simultaneously endotracheal pressure was recorded (B, lower tracing), the inflation during artificial ventilation being represented by an upward deflection. The upward potentials occurred only during inflations of the lungs.

This pattern is represented in the lower tracing of the histogram (A) by spikes corresponding to black squares (which indicate inflations). The time base of the histogram is one-third of respiratory cycle (corresponding to inflation).

In control conditions (left part of A), this spike activity occurred only during inflations of the lungs but not during all of them (the average discharge per second being indicated by the number on top of histogram).

During coronary occlusion (middle part of A), the discharge was still inflation-locked, but its association with the respiratory cycle became more regular, a spike corresponding practically to each inflation. This regularity decreased at the release of coronary occlusion (right part of A).

After vagotomy (C and D), likely to interrupt most of pulmonary afferents, the inflation-locked pattern of fiber discharge was lost: conversely, the reflex excitation elicited by coronary artery occlusion was unmodified.

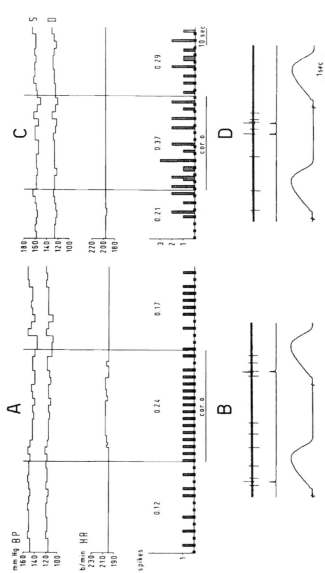

Figure 48: Effects of coronary occlusion (cor.o.) on a sympathetic fiber discharge. Of the two fibers simultaneously recorded in B and D (upper tracings), that with a predominantly negative potential (upward deflection) has been selected for calculation of the histograms in A and C. Histogram time base is one-third of respiratory cycle (black squares indicate inflations). In B and D, upper tracing is cathode-ray oscilloscope record of fiber discharge; middle tracing is polygraph record of pulses triggered by each upward action potential; lower tracing is polygraph record of endotracheal pressure (inflation upwards). A and B: before vagotomy; C and D: after vagotomy. Note relationship of fiber discharge with inflation (A and B) lost after vagotomy (C and D).

This experiment provides an example of synchronization between two processes. In fact, the rise in sympathetic activity induced by coronary occlusion occurs only during a specific phase of ventilation (i.e. all other phases are forbidden). This relationship is nonlinear, because if it were linear the two processes should not appear phase-locked but independent of each other.

Frequency tracking locus

In order to obtain a more quantitative assessment of phase relationship and locking ratio of a nonlinear interaction between two different variables, *ad hoc* tools are necessary.

One of such tools is represented by the frequency tracking locus (Kitney and Bignall 1993) that can be better explained by the experiment of Figure 49.

Sympathetic impulse activity was recorded from a multifiber preparation, obtained in a decerebrate unanesthetized cat artificially ventilated (Montano et al. 1992). Ventilatory cycles are indicated by the dotted line (Figure 49, a, b, and c) and the artificial positive pressure ventilation is considered as a *forcing input*.

Sympathetic activity was analogically counted in temporal frames of 20 msec, A/D converted, and filtered at 1 Hz in order to eliminate cardiac rhythmicity. Both ventilatory and sympathetic signals were sampled once per cardiac cycle (approximately 3Hz in cats), in order to obtain their synchronous beat-to-beat variability series. Sympathetic activity is considered as a *forced output* and is indicated by the continuous line in Figure 49 (a, b and c).

The key for comprehending the graph represented in *d*, referring to the tracing *a* (control conditions), is quite simple. Considering in *a* the second ventilatory cycle (from the left), it appears that it is preceded by a sympathetic burst with a phase greater than π (i.e. half period). All the subsequent sympathetic bursts display a similar phase relationship: by convention phase rotation is measured counterclockwise and is represented in *d* as the phase of the individual vectors, remaining relatively constant at ~230°. However the plot also indicates the ratio between the amplitude of the sympathetic burst and of ventilation as the length of the vector. This relationship corresponding to a 1:1 dynamics, as each ventilatory cycle is accompanied by a sympathetic burst, further characterizes the mechanisms involved in generating synchronous HF components in the respective power spectra.

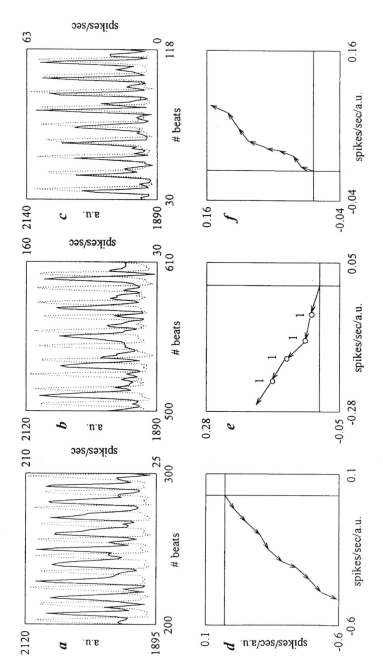

Figure 49: Top panels: superposition of ventilatory (dotted line) and sympathetic (continuous line) series; bottom panels: corresponding patterns of frequency tracking locus. Control conditions: *a* and *d*; sympathetic excitation (obtained with inferior vena cava occlusion): *b* and *e*; sympathetic inhibition (obtained with aortic constriction): *c* and *f*.

From subsequent and different control conditions, a sympathetic excitation was obtained by reducing venous return with inferior vena cava occlusion (*b*). The sympathetic bursts become closer to the following ventilatory peaks and, consequently, the phase is reduced to less than π in the frequency tracking locus (*e*). Moreover, not all ventilatory cycles are accompanied by a sympathetic burst (b): the small open circles (*e*) denote this absence. The relationship corresponds in this case to a 1:2 dynamics. The interpretation of this phenomenon has to consider the presence of both LF and HF components in the power spectrum of sympathetic discharge variability (see Figure 27): hence it is likely that during 1:2 dynamics the LF component is locked at half the frequency of ventilation, while HF becomes unlocked (Porta et al. 1996).

Finally, during a sympathetic inhibition obtained by inc⸗ sing arterial pressure with aortic constriction (*c*), the sympathetic bursts are still closer to the following ventilatory cycles. Hence, in the frequency tracking locus the phase is further reduced, while the relationship corresponds again to a 1:1 dynamics (*f*).

This experiment thus shows that complex oscillatory events (LF and HF) can be locked to the same *forcing input* with different modes. However there are also conditions in which the same oscillatory phenomena interact only very weakly.

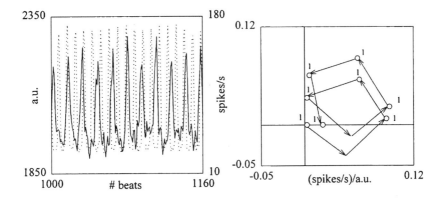

Figure 50: Left panel: superposition of ventilatory (dotted line) and sympathetic (continuous line) series; right panel: corresponding pattern of frequency tracking locus indicating a quasi-periodic dynamics. See text. (From Porta et al. 1996, with permission).

In the case of Figure 50, referring to an experiment similar to the one previously described, the relationship between ventilatory peaks and sympathetic bursts changes continuously (left panel). This is quantified by the phase rotation occurring in the frequency tracking locus (right panel).

These few examples should indicate quite clearly that different *patterns* can be individuated and classified with relatively simple tools which, however, are capable of disclosing the complexity hidden in apparently similar phenomena.

INFORMATION DOMAIN

"The concepts of regularity, synchronization and coordination are central in biology and medicine as they are strongly linked to thé information exchange among (sub)systems composing the whole organism and, therefore, to its organization" (Porta 1998; Porta et al. 2000).

In this perspective, capturing the information content from the time series of biological signals is not only an affair of researcher's curiosity but a key for understanding. I have already anticipated in *Chapter 3* that the widespread distribution among neural structures of LF and HF spectral components suggests their link with an information code. In the case of *patterns* the attempt is to define some of their properties that might also belong to an information code.

Definition of regularity
This definition, like the others that will follow, is non formal, that is, intuitive (Porta 1998).

The concept of *regularity* is intended to characterize the dynamics of one signal. It can be defined as the degree of recurrence of a specific pattern (waveform) exhibited by the signal. When a pattern – even the most complex one – is fully repetitive, the signal is periodic and this corresponds to the maximal level of *regularity*.

If the pattern occurs repetitively in the signal dynamics but other features are also present (trends, different waveforms, transient episodes, irregular oscillations) *regularity* is reduced. If repetitive patterns are absent, *regularity* is null.

Different levels of *regularity* correspond to different levels of information carried by the signal. A strictly periodical signal is completely predictable from its own past samples. Therefore, the information carried by the ongoing signal is null. Fully irregular dynamics (i.e. white noise) is unpredictable and its information content is very high. A series with some level of *regularity* is neither completely unpredictable nor fully predictable, thus carrying some amount of information.

In experimental terms, *regularity* is measured by means of functions that quantify the *entropy* rate of a process, corresponding to the amount of information carried by the last sample of the series when a portion of the previous samples is known. These functions exploit the conditional probability to assess whether the series is more or less predictable from its own past. Thus *regularity* is the inverse of *entropy*: if the series is regular (i.e. strictly periodical and completely predictable) the *entropy* rate is zero. If the series is a white noise (i.e. completely irregular and totally unpredictable) the *entropy* rate is high. The *entropy* rate of series with some level of *regularity* is between these two extremes.

Several functions have been proposed to approximate the entropy rate of short segments of data and to derive indexes of *regularity*. A widely used index is the *approximate entropy* proposed by Pincus (1991).

More recently, Porta et al (1998) proposed a new function referred to as corrected conditional entropy (CCE). The main advantage of this function is that the derived index of *regularity* is obtained without setting *a priori* the embedding dimension of the reconstructed phase space (i.e., the number of previous samples used to predict).

When applied to short data sequences (around 250-300 samples) the CCE exhibits a minimum and the smaller is its value the more regular is the series.

An example of *regularity* measurement using the CCE is shown in Figure 51. The analysis is performed on three time series of RR variability recorded from the same normal subject. In control conditions, the tachogram (*a*) and its power spectrum (*b*) correspond to a CCE that presents a minimum level around 1, indicating some level of regularity. During passive head-up tilt, the tachogram (*d*) and its power spectrum (*e*) undergo the usual changes, while the minimum of CCE (f) is clearly decreased to around 0.6. Thus tilt was able to increase both the LF oscillation and the regularity of heart period series. Conversely, controlled respiration at 20 breaths per minute (*g*), although capable of sharpening the HF component in the power spectrum (*h*), does not increase the regularity as it does not modify the minimum of CCE (*i*).

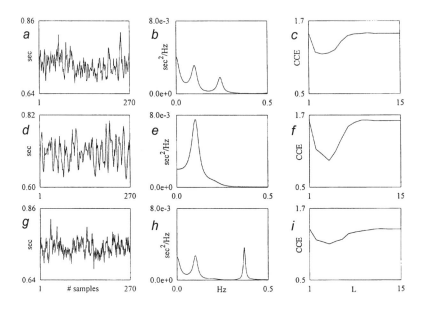

Figure 51:   RR series (left panels), autospectra (middle panels) and corrected conditional entropy – CCE (right panels) obtained from a normal subject in control conditions (*a, b, c*), during passive head-up tilt (*d, e, f*) and during controlled respiration at 20 breaths/min (*g, h, i*).   See text. (From Porta et al. 1997, with permission).

Interestingly, it has been recently reported that healthy ageing is associated with RR interval dynamics characterized by higher regularity (Pikkujämsä et al. 1999).

The search for regularity can also furnish interesting observations in pathophysiological conditions.   In Figure 52 the same approach is applied to recordings obtained from a normal subject (A) and from a patient with advanced heart failure (B).   In the normal subject, as described in Figure 51, the sympathetic activation during tilt is accompanied by an increased *regularity*.

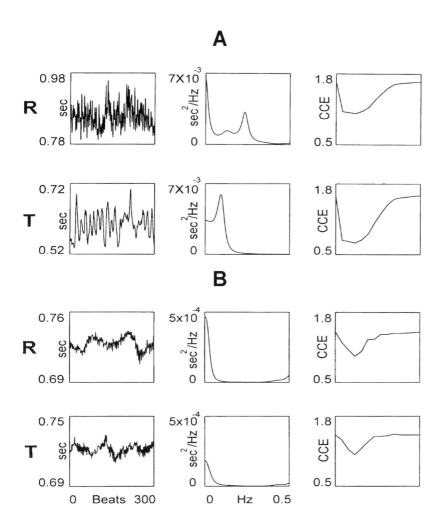

Figure 52: RR series (left panels), autospectra (middle panels) and CCE (right panels). A: normal subject; B: patient with advanced heart failure; both studied in resting conditions (R) and during head-up tilt (T). (From Guzzetti et al. 1995, unpublished observations).

In the heart failure patient the power spectrum, in resting conditions, presents only a VLF component as already described (Guzzetti et al. 1995) but some regularity is indicated by CCE minimum. However, during tilt both power spectrum and CCE remain practically unchanged.

Thus, this is another way to substantiate the notion that neural regulatory mechanisms become largely inoperative in patients with advanced heart failure.

Definition of synchronization

The concept of *regularity* can be generalized when two signals or a set of signals are contemporaneously present. This generalization leads to the concepts of *synchronization* and *coordination* (Porta 1998).

Synchronization is intended to characterize the relationship between two interacting signals. It can be defined as the degree of recurrence of a *pattern* involving the two signals. If the *pattern* is repetitive, the two signals are strongly coupled and the information carried by the two signals is not larger than the one carried by either signal. If no repetitive *pattern* is present, the two signals are independent (*synchronization* is null) and the information carried by the two signals is the sum of the information carried by each of them. Intermediate levels of *synchronization* are found when a sliding coupling between the two signals is present (i.e. when their link changes in time).

Synchronization is assessed by means of the minimum of the *uncoupling function* (UF), that calculates with *entropy* rates the minimum amount of independent information (i.e. the information carried by one signal that cannot be derived from the other) (Porta et al. 1999). Thus also in this case, the maximal *synchronization* corresponds to the minimum of the *uncoupling function*.

In the case of Figure 53, *synchronization* between respiratory movements (dotted line) and RR changes (continuous line) is assessed during spontaneous respiration (A) and during metronome breathing at 10 breaths per minute (B). With this latter maneuver *synchronization* is clearly increased, independently of the concomitant levels of *regularity*, characterizing either signal.

This approach can be applied to pathophysiology as well. In the case of Figure 54 *synchronization* between the changes in RR (dotted line) and RT (continuous line) intervals (Porta et al. 1999) is estimated. It is a well-established notion that changes in RR determine parallel variations in RT interval, implying that these two variables are intrinsically correlated. Thus it is not surprising to find in a normal subject (A) a high level of *synchronization*. However, what was surprising was to observe that this *synchronization* is practically lost in a patient after myocardial infarction (B), a phenomenon that could not be expected on the basis of other measurements.

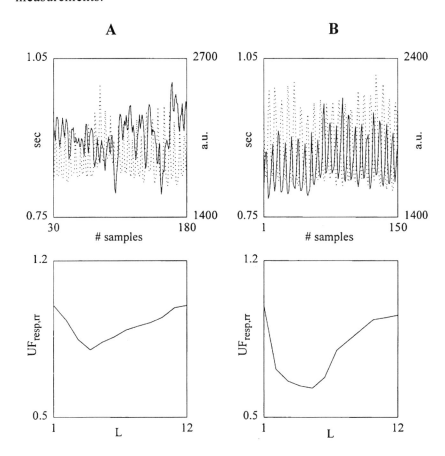

Figure 53: Superposition of beat-to-beat changes of variability series of both ventilatory movements (dotted line) and RR intervals (continuous line) recorded from a normal subject during spontaneous respiration (A) and during metronome breathing at 10 acts per minute. See text. (From Porta 1998, unpublished observations).

Definition of coordination

The concept of *coordination* is intended to characterize the level of cooperativeness among a set of variables involved in a complex and specific task (Porta et al. 2000). It can be defined as the degree of recurrence of a *pattern* common to all involved variables. A set of coordinated signals is characterized by a large number of repetitions of a common *pattern* and by a low information content. Conversely, a set of independent signals exhibits no repetitive structure and carries a large amount of information.

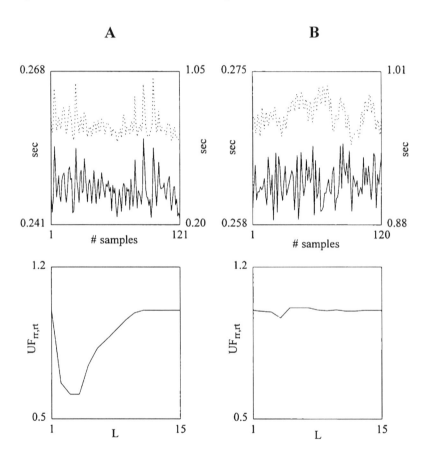

Figure 54: Superposition of beat-to-beat changes of variability series of both RR (dotted line) and RT (solid line) intervals recorded in a normal subject (A) and in a patient after myocardial infarction (B). See text. (From Porta et al. 1999, with permission).

A clear example of *coordination* is represented by animal locomotion, which is generated and controlled by central patterns capable of producing coordinated rhythmic outputs. Each coordinated *pattern* corresponds to a different gait (e.g. walk, trot, gallop). A brief loss of *coordination* among the signals occurs during a transition from one gait to another. The stable loss of *coordination* among the central *pattern* generators impairs locomotion, even though single movements might be preserved.

Patterns and symbols

Pattern recognition can be based on quite different approaches. For instance, under the hypothesis that the sources of HRV might also be discontinuous and localized in specific segments of the sequences, it has been proposed that such sequences might be organized, like sentences are (Roach et al. 1999). In short there would be a lexicon of recurrent similarly shaped transient structures like words, and each word would have a characteristic physiological basis (Le Pape et al. 1997). Roach et al (1999) coined the term "*lexon*" to refer to some meaningful transient structures in heart period sequences. The brief tachycardia (named "burst") that occurs at the initiation of exercise was considered an appropriate *lexon*. Interestingly, bursts that were morphologically similar were induced when subjects rolled themselves from supine to lateral decubitus positions and viceversa. Accordingly, in 24-hour Holter recordings from healthy subjects about 120 bursts were detected, morphologically similar to those induced with appropriate maneuvers.

A remarkable pathophysiological application of *pattern* recognition was recently reported by Schmidt et al (1999). These Authors observed that a single ventricular premature beat (VPB) was usually followed by an early acceleration and subsequent deceleration of sinus rhythm – a pattern that was termed *heart-rate turbulence*. Two numerical parameters quantified this turbulence, termed *turbulence onset* and *slope*. Positive percent values of *turbulence onset* corresponded to sinus rhythm deceleration after a VBP, while negative values indicated sinus rhythm acceleration (i.e. the selected *pattern*). The values of *turbulence slope* were expressed in msec per RR interval, corresponding to the maximum positive slope of a regression line over any sequence of five subsequent sinus rhythm RR intervals.

In patients recovering from myocardial infarction *heart rate turbulence* after VPB was found to be a very potent risk stratifier with optimal dichotomies at 0 for *turbulence onset* and 2.5 msec per RR interval for *turbulence slope*. For instance, the relative hazard of the combination of both abnormal parameters (i.e. *onset* ≥ 0 and *slope* ≤ 2.5 msec) was 3.2. This figure was greater than any other obtained with usual risk predictors: as an example, the relative hazard of an EF < 30% was 2.9.

The Authors advanced various hypotheses in order to explain the *heart-rate turbulence* including "ventriculophasic" phenomena. An alternative hypothesis is that this interesting *pattern* might rather reflect the sympathetic burst following a VPB (Lombardi et al. 1989) and a subsequent vagal rebound in a brief oscillation of sympathovagal balance. If this was the case, the reported prognostic value of a decreased *turbulence* would represent a remarkable example of the pathophysiological significance of the reduction of cardiovascular neurally-mediated oscillations. As to the involved mechanisms, a closed-loop schema would also in this case be essential. In fact, a reduced heart rate response might be caused by a decreased cardiac responsiveness to neural modulation and/or might also be the source of an abnormal afferent input to the centers, and hence of an altered reflex modulation.

However, these studies should suffice to indicate that the search for *patterns* seems to be a highly promising perspective, quite new and quite old as it often occurs in science.

Chance

The study of linear and nonlinear dynamics and, more in general, the post elaboration of a variability signal has the main purpose of extracting the information content imbedded in any sequence. The more we learn the less is left to chance.

On the other hand, the appraisal of casuality also requires adequate cultural and psychological tools. This is true not only in science but in all domains pertaining to human condition. We fear chance and we are attracted by it.

Stéphane Mallarmé wrote *"un coup de dés jamais n'abolira le hasard"*. This may be translated as *a throw of dice will never cast the hazard*. Hazard being an arab word (*azzahr*) that means dice. Thus circling goes on.

Chapter 6
THE NECESSARY APICAL PRINCIPLE IN SCIENCE AND MEDICINE

The whole scientific endeavor makes sense only if it is primarily aimed at improving human condition. It has often been so, but not always – and now less than ever. In such a case, some ethical rules should also be mandatory but, again, they have been too often ignored. These *a priori* requirements would be clearly reflected by an overall neutrality of science, meaning a permanent and fruitful debate in the absence of polarized manipulation of knowledge. But science has never been neutral. And its manipulation is nowadays a business of enormous proportions.

This *Chapter* does not have the foolish purpose of analyzing *"the structure of scientific revolutions"* (Kuhn 1970), but only of wishfully contributing to a state of ethical consciousness, fortunately quite diffused, for which every single line of scientific writing could be an occasion to precisely reinforce a project for a more neutral science.

The control of science, different from manipulation, has been in the past even more devastating, the examples of Galileo Galilei or Giordano Bruno being of everlasting power. However replacing Popes with business has created new problems.

Through aggregates of concepts, scientific societies and international journals quite strong theories often arise that, when conjugated to economical profit, become an almost insurmountable barrier against a new way of thinking. On the other hand *"philosophers of science have repeatedly demonstrated that more than one theoretical construction can always be placed upon a given collection of data"* (Kuhn 1970).

Thus, it is the absence of debate that often reveals a scientific poverty. However, nowadays time runs fast and what may appear as a stable control over a theory is continuously jeopardized by the anarchic courage of myriads of people searching for the opposite (end of

Chapter 4), by nonlinear interactions and hence by chance (end of *Chapter 5*). Thus in the end, the boat is again at open sea.

In this perspective a control of science according to criteria (Lakatos 1978) that may be worthy of respect, rich in substance but independent of scientific practice and in the hands of the non scientific society, becomes unnecessary and perhaps dangerous. Simply, while doing their best to counteract this process, scientists have to learn to bear the sadness deriving from the ubiquitous shows featuring manipulation of science.

In these few pages, I shall try to visit (Malliani 1999b) some of our daily problems in research and in medicine, that reflect the interaction of rational and nonrational determinants, purely scientific logics, human-oriented and profit-oriented tendencies and other facets of a complexity different from that already analyzed, in the hope of finding at least a thin ethical Ariadne's thread.

Transparency

In clinical medicine, the practice of informed consent is finally growing. Controlled clinical trials cannot be carried out without it. But, in fact, how truly informed is the consent? What has the human cost for placebo been? Would a physician treat himself with a double-blind approach?

We know quite well that, methodologically, an experiment (or trial) requires controlled conditions. Yet, often, these experiments are quite costly from a human point of view. Moreover, trials are becoming of utmost importance. Too many people consider trials supreme research rather than a mere application. We must try to develop improved observational methods for evaluating therapeutic effectiveness, so that perhaps, one day, the placebo will be obsolete and the thousands of enrolled patients unnecessary.

Yet, one of the greatest threats to the neutrality of science, which has emerged during the last decades and which is growing exponentially throughout the world, is the conflict of interests.

In the same hands one can find economic links, as many as possible, with the industry, the government of trials and of scientific societies, the organization of countless meetings, international journals publishing editorials, and the pen for writing guidelines that correspond to how public and private money will be spent. This scientific-industrial complex, in spite of its widespread germination, has the structure of a bunker.

I know that there are always good reasons for reality to happen, however, they are not necessarily the best reasons. From a scientific point of view, this state of affairs has nothing to do with the ethics of progress and of communication. From an industrial point of view, it is amazing that aggressive, multinational companies have not yet realized that having these bunkers as a common denominator is a fearful and short-sighted strategy. The most patent result obtained by obeying these lobbies of advisors has been to homogenize the scientific profile of different drugs. Indeed what is known about a drug is largely a consequence of the models that have been used for its study. Similar experimental models rarely produce new perspectives. Thus the scientific imagination becomes trivial and is usually replaced by a harder commercial competition, often open to corruption. Meanwhile progressive company mergers, implying unemployed people, are on the horizon.

In my view, transparency for a scientist willing to contribute to the search for new therapies means believing in one hypothesis, belonging to one team, following one single path, with its related risks and benefits, and not all possible simultaneous enterprises, floating without personal risks on this ocean of money. For those playing the game it should be mandatory to keep out of editorials and guidelines covering the specific matter. So far, it seems unlikely that subtracting their expertise will jeopardize public health.

An international code of conduct is highly needed – which would immediately produce a cascade of enjoyable effects among which more innovative scientific findings, better distributed resources and less boring meetings, in the absence of ritual repetitions of often precedented novelties.

To provide an example of minimal importance, but that I know quite well, an invited speech on positive feedback reflexes has never been hosted during one of the thousands of international meetings on arterial hypertension, that have instead devoted much more than the due time to baroreceptors and negative feedback mechanisms. Thus, instead of facing the provocation of the new experimental findings and their soundness, the polarized establishment has also neglected, to take a strictly correlated example, the fact that the hypertensive crises that can be triggered by an abdominal stimulation in quadriplegic patients are difficult to explain on the basis of negative feedback mechanisms. So, these crises being outside the main market for their short duration and for the relatively restricted number of patients, their pathogenesis that might have had a pivotal conceptual role has remained a physiological affair.

Myriads of similar examples act as litmus paper in signaling a pH far from neutrality. In addition, it is in my opinion far from certain that science, at times, does not lose some common sense. Still using the example of arterial hypertension, large trials can find significant differences of less than 5 mmHg, thus influencing classifications and prescriptions. But it is well-known that direct and indirect arterial pressure measurements can differ by more than 10 mmHg, even in the most expert hands, and that these values oscillate continuously even in resting conditions. Thus we use general figures that cannot be soundly assessed at individual level. This scientific paradox should be much more considered when facing the classification and treatment of individual patients and should stimulate a more critical and less integralistic attitude from the experts with their guidelines.

However, in the long run a decent barycentre is always attained in science and some neutrality is reconquered. These manipulations are even more unbearable in clinical medicine, because any divergence from the best we may accomplish is made up of human condition.

Physicians somehow represent the transmission belt connecting science products and patients needs in a relationship that can never be totally neutral or equal, and thus has to respond to ethical rules.

"*What is unique today is the unprecedented power of medical knowledge and the enormity of the potential profit to be made through its use. Given the pervasive spread of commercialism throughout the health care system, the obligation to use medical power with ethical constraint is more urgent than ever* (Pellegrino and Relman 1999)".

The ethical needs

Ethos is an ancient Greek word that means habit, custom, or behavior. Different people and civilizations obviously had different conceptualizations of ethics and, therefore, it is likely that the science of morality will never provide a system that is valid for all and forever.

By now ethics has stopped being a Kantian doctrine of "*categorical imperatives*" and more so, according to Hegel, a philosophy of history. It nowadays rather appears as a complex and critical point of reference, based on the most different experiences, from mainly pragmatic to intimate and barely definable ones – a vast territory open to individual and social dialogue. These permanent dynamics seem to neutralize the fear for future disasters comparable to some of the past, which on their occurrence – think of the Crusades or of racial persecutions – were even ascribed an ethical value.

In this arena values and rules acquire and lose their structure, and here is where we approach a relevant question: why does a man – a *medicus* - try to help someone else? In his novel *La Peste* (*The Plague*), published in 1943, Albert Camus has expressed some of the greatest thoughts on this human attitude .

In addition to pestilence being an obvious metaphor of war - leading to similar confinement, helplessness, profound darkness and fatalism - the key of the novel somehow consists in the equivalence of different points of view in front of the same absurdity. A physician, Dr. Rieux, struggles beyond his strength because he cannot get used to seeing people die. But the true enigma, and the simplest human solution, is embodied by Tarrou. He is not a doctor, but he struggles as much as if he were, or even more. One day, asked by Dr. Rieux about what drives him to behave this way, he answers "*la compréhension*", comprehension.

What is comprehension? The Latin word *comprehendere* means to take in, to grasp, so comprehension becomes the act of grasping with the intellect, and the attitude of incorporating becomes the possibility of being understood. In short it opens the door to reciprocity.

Hopefully the voice *I ought* will never disappear. What is needed is to reconcile this aspect of the inner supreme moral law with the needs of individuals and those of society. Medicine becomes a tragic theater when a choice is necessary between the needs of an individual person and those of the society. A man, a doctor, is alone when he has to pass that *porte étroite*, that narrow door, when a decision has to be taken. You do that, you don't do that. The rest are details.

The *theory of need* is probably an acceptable and updated substitute for a castle of *a priori* duties. Its complexity is extreme, taking as an example the work by Agnès Heller (1974). In our context, to clarify some terms, a few allusions will suffice.

The ensemble of needs is highly heterogeneous, though there are two main categories. The first includes natural needs necessary to any existence, such as the need of food, of sexual activity, of a tolerable temperature. As a doctor I would also consider a necessary need the interruption of an unbearable pain. The second category includes needs that are primarily human and socially determined, such as cultural activity, self-realization, affective and moral attributes. These are qualitative needs. However social aggregation also induces purely quantitative needs, that one may rather call *wants* and that can grow indefinitely and are potentially alienating. The sovereign example is the endless accumulation of wealth. It is curious that for this same theory, the true wealth is spare time and nothing more.

As doctors we deal continuously not only with the natural but also with the social needs of our patients. And in addition, now more than ever, we have to attempt to reconcile these individual needs with those of society. The luminous sentence *"the highest object of the human need is the other human being"* is sometimes more a trust than a must, and this terrible paradox is often the hallmark of the unhappiness of a physician. But it is also a trigger for honesty. And as Dr. Rieux says: *"I don't know about honesty generally speaking, but in my case I know it consists in doing my profession"*.

The structure of medicine

"Medicine is not a science but a learned profession, deeply rooted in a number of sciences and charged with the obligation to apply them for man's benefit", is how W. McDermott (1971) described it. However, looking more deeply in its scientific attributes, it appears that a matrix of at least two dimensions is required to display the structure of scientific knowledge. According to Blois (1988), in a hierarchical schema of sciences, near the bottom there are atomic physics and other hard or exact sciences, where strict laws express the generalization inferred from experimental data. At the top there are the sciences regarded as soft, or inexact. At the bottom, it is believed to be true that positive and negative electric charges attract each other; at the top, it is believed to be true that loneliness can cause depression. *"Hence, the problem in medical reasoning arises from an uncertainty of how to combine all our observational data, which may range from the chemistry and physics of physiologic processes to ethical issues and subtle and vagal clinical impressions"*.

Taking Blois' example of a patient with Wilson's disease, the hierarchical levels include at the atomic level the disturbance of the copper, and above the consequences on biopolymers, on cells, on organs, on physiological systems, on the patient as a whole including his malaise, bizarre behavior, bipolar psychoses. An internist – my own vest as a physician – has to possess the ability of vertical reasoning and has to develop sufficient knowledge of all involved horizontal layers. Even in terms of approach, while the reductionistic models are essential at basic and intermediate levels, an observational strategy is necessary when the complexity cannot be cut into pieces.

Great courage is needed to ask the question: with an asymmetrical and discontinuous knowledge, how can internists be useful to their patients?

Surprisingly, the answer is quite simple. Inasmuch as human beings do not simply function but live, insofar as the whole individual is much more than the sum of his organs, inasmuch as there is a difference between complicated structures, like a watch needing to be disassembled in order to be better understood, and complex realities like pain that cannot be simplified, internists should not feel to be just remnants but rather pupils at the school of complexity. This should not dismiss their gratitude for the innumerable reductionistic achievements.

Life, disease, death are complex entities and complex is the physician's task too. A great method is necessary to face the uncertainty that grows with complexity. The method which is needed is, in fact, a federation of methods. The method required for the acquisition of new basic notions, or for experimental medicine (which is still the best Academy), is different from the one needed to interpret human behavior. Thus it is not surprising that the so-called medical competence is based on the continuous pursuit of ever-changing concepts and views.

Partly related to this growing complexity, one has to realize that the patient-physician relationship is at risk of an unprecedented mutation, the consequences of which cannot be foreseen.

In a brilliant viewpoint Herman (1998) wrote that *"nostalgia, defined as a longing for something far away or long ago, permeates our attempts to redefine the relationship between patient and doctor in the light of social evolution and recent developments. This longing suggests dissatisfaction with the present and, perhaps, a conviction that things used to be better"*. Obviously there is no sound evidence that we should be nostalgic for yesterday. In addition, we cannot in any circumstance stem the tide of change in the society in which we live. And yet the strain is increasing. In terms of non linear dynamics and chaos theory, we might, independently of nostalgia, reach a point of so-called bifurcation.

The lost art of healing

This is the title of a book by Bernard Lown (1996) in which he writes: *"I am persuaded that touching a patient provides advantages to the internist, as compared with the psychiatrist who sits removed and merely listens. Touching is a means for gaining significant insights. Frequently the conversation at a first interview is impersonal. The relationship with the patient often alters dramatically after the physical examination. The remoteness dissipates, supplanted by comfortable easy-flowing conversation. Material that was neither divulged nor suspected emerges without much probing. Questioning is no longer resented. A stranger a few minutes earlier opens up with intimacies usually earned only through long and trusting friendship".*

This is the kind of doctor a patient would like to meet, the patient being simply a fellow human in need of help. Each human being is unique with a life that is, *per se*, enormously complex, and each patient has the need to have his uniqueness be recognized. For this reason, the doctor has to stay with and listen to his patient.

The following are words by Wilfred Trotter, a great English neurosurgeon:

"... As long as medicine is an art, its chief and characteristic instrument must be human faculty. We come therefore to the very practical question of what aspects of human faculty it is necessary for the good doctor to cultivate... The first to be named must always be the power of attention, of giving one's whole mind to the patient without the interposition of oneself. It sounds simple but only the very greatest doctors ever fully attain it. It is an active process and not either mere resigned listening or even politely waiting until you can interrupt. Disease often tells its secrets in a casual parenthesis..." (as quoted by Smith 1988).

Reciprocal education

Osler early in this century (as quoted by Atchley 1967) cited Galen as saying, *"He cures most successfully in whom the people have the greatest confidence".*

It is likely that a sympathetic and discerning history has always provided the first and most important step as the patient and doctor come to know each other. Communication on the emotional level is a basic requirement for initiating relationship at other levels. However, a firm foundation requires communication on an intellectual level. Here, reciprocity is crucial. A doctor has to become a teacher and an attentive listener to his patient's ideas. In this communication, the level of mutual integrity is so vital to be given almost top priority. That is, a physician should always admit his mistakes. As Horton, editor of

Lancet, recently wrote (1999) *"the issue is not whether errors occur, but what doctors learn from them... Patients are more likely to be reassured by a profession that faces up to its mistakes than by one that buries them"*.

In brief, we should try to take care of others as we ourselves would like to be taken care of. It might appear banal and yet, sometimes, it is almost utopian. Avalanches of tests, sometimes invasive, are often performed for the sake of thoroughness in the best case, or for economical purposes, in the worst case. Accordingly, drugs and doses should be similar to those that physicians would take themselves, while considering also the quality of life.

Ivan Illich (1975) began his book *"Medical nemesis"* with the statement that *"the medical establishment has become the major threat to health"*. Part of this fear was surely an anticipation of the progressive loss of reciprocity.

On the other hand, Skrabanek (1998) has stressed that: *"Medicine is an authoritarian institution which feels threatened when its dogmas are exposed as unfounded"*.

Not surprisingly, *"problems with the quality of health care can be categorized as overuse, underuse and misuse"* (Bodenheimer 1999). Overuse of operations or diagnostic procedures has been largely documented. As for underuse, in the USA, the quality of care within hospitals has been found to be inferior for blacks and uninsured. Concerning misuse, it has been written that 180.000 people die each year in the USA partly as a result of injuries, such as adverse drug reactions, caused by physicians (Bodenheimer 1999). Other countries are only different in not attempting similar surveys.

Fortunately, a vibrant movement to improve the quality of health is springing up in several countries. Despite its ups and downs, a human desire will always exist to do the right thing.

In short, until man understands why ego is *I* and not *thou* , any encounter must be reciprocal. In fact, even *I* and *me* do not fully coincide: usually, during the night while *I* is dreaming, *me* is sleeping. What we have gained or lost by being *I* and *me* instead of *thou* is an enigma.

The final goal of medicine

What is the final goal of medicine? Perhaps the attempt to guarantee a good, natural death (in the etymological sense of *euthanasia*) when, at the end of a good life, it might be possible to leave the table as sated guests. Sometimes death is an event; other times it is a path. When a patient is nearing death from an illness that is progressive and unrelenting, the word *terminal* is often used. It is a harsh word, better suited for a computer. Usually, poor people become *terminal* earlier than rich people. The Head of a government can die, after months of illness, without having been *terminal*: in this business-based society, one wonders whether *terminal* means that the patient has *terminated*, has stopped being productive, as it occurs when the whole medical machinery cannot invent anything decent any longer. We know that it is not always so, but we know that it can be so. The point is that too often *terminal* patients are abandoned.

Pietas, a beautiful Latin word that is not piety as it is more lay, and that is not compassion as it is more reciprocal without pretending to be love, should pervade a physician when he is close to the mystery of death.

A relevant question is how many human beings, without being ill, are in fact considered *terminal* for years and years? This is the case with the mentally disabled, with heavy drug addicts, and with poor, old people, to mention just a few. I am not sure that this is only a matter of economic resources. It is a question of civilization.

The role of physicians

It is my firm belief, and that of history, that a physician's role involves everything dealing with the human condition. Doctors on the road have attempted practically everything. Less notoriously than Albert Schweitzer in Lambarene, thousands of them have risked or lost their lives during the war, to be on the field, or in peace, to study an infectious disease. Not so many years ago the International Physicians for the Prevention of Nuclear War had a tremendous cultural impact on making the Heads of nuclear powers understand that a nuclear war would not be limited and would result in the last epidemic for human beings. Nowadays "*Médecins sans frontières*", "*Emergency*" and numerous other organizations are present where many tragedies occur.

And it is a marvellous coincidence that on the very day I am writing these words the newspapers report the award of the 1999 Nobel Peace Prize to "*Médecins sans frontières*".

In terms of wishful thinking I expect, in the near future, to see physicians much more involved in many of our daily problems, such as the pollution that is destroying our urban areas, or the pacific genocide acting through the political and criminal organization of the drug market.

Or more involved in caring for the aged. When an old human being is sent to retirement and becomes unproductive, if he is poor, if he has no family around, when the plug is pulled out and the power collapses, anything occurring to him has nothing to do with the dignity that society should confer to the end of human life. For too many years we have been talking much more about embryos than about old people. We are constantly intimated not to abandon a dog, but we have no problem in forgetting about an old person.

Or more involved in facing the problem that every two seconds a child somewhere dies for reasons related to malnutrition. For those of us who live in the northern hemisphere, eating less food would be the most effective way to prevent cardiovascular and other diseases. For those living in the southern part of the planet, eating more food would produce even better effects. It is a strange paradox for the global village, in which the majority of the population has never made a telephone call.

It is hypocritical to think, as many people do, that when we shall know more we shall do better - the leitmotiv for requesting money for research. We know already enough to do much better. If we did so, then we might deserve to ask for money for research.

The reason why I say this is not only Tarrou's comprehension in *The Plague*. It is more selfish. We do, we overdo, but we are less and less happy. Everything improves, and yet we are progressively more and more mentally disturbed and full of nostalgia. Our children fear the future. They feel that it will be out of their control. Only an ethical project for the future can address the many problems we have created. Medicine, so close to nature and human needs, could be a fundamental catalyst to develop the immense consciousness required to find a way out.

The way out

In Franz Kafka short story *"A report to an Academy"*, a man explains to their Excellencies the Academicians how, five years earlier, he was a monkey and how he became a man. He was wounded, captured, and entrapped in a cage that was much too small for him. He realized that there was no way out. Yet, he had to find a way out. He never hoped for freedom, merely a way out, in the most common sense of the word. Hence he stopped being a monkey. He learned to spit, he learned to speak, and this was his way out, into the world of mankind. As a consequence, he was now speaking in front of their Excellencies.

If an entrapped monkey could find a way out, hopefully an entrapped man would at least try. Obviously, we should learn to spit and speak in a different way, just as a monkey would imagine men should do. Otherwise?

So Jove said to the other gods: "See now, how men lay blame upon us gods for what is after all nothing but their own folly" (Odyssey, Book I, translated by Samuel Butler).

Paraphrasing again, *human beings often call destiny their folly.*

APPENDIX

for the general reader

This appendix is intended to facilitate the reading for those who are not particularly acquainted with the study of neural mechanisms regulating cardiovascular function.

Feedback schema

All feedback control systems have certain features in common (Houk and Henneman 1974). A block diagram with these features clearly identified provides the best guide to outline the regulatory mechanisms. Figure 1 illustrates a double control system, to be analyzed separately. The lower half of the Figure corresponds to a negative feedback mechanism. The *controlled system*, corresponding to the cardiovascular (CV) system, has an input, represented by the arrow, that can be varied by the *controller* represented by the central nervous system (CNS). This input interacts with external influences called *disturbances* and produces changes in the *output* corresponding to the variable to be controlled, that is arterial pressure. The baroreceptors are one example of transducers, that is a sensitive device placed where it can measure the actual output of the *controlled system*. It converts this measurement into a *feedback signal*, which is transmitted to an error detector. Here it is compared with the *reference signal*, which is the primary input of the entire feedback system. Since the *reference signal* dictates a desired output and the *feedback signal* measures the actual output, the difference computed at the error detector is called *error signal*. Applied to the *reference signal*, that is to the primary *controller*, the *error signal* alters the input to the *controlled* system so as to reduce the amount of error. The actual output is thus brought close to the output specified by the *reference signal*. This compensatory action is the aim of a *negative feedback* system, hence the sign *minus*.

Conversely, the upper part of the Figure corresponds to a positive feedback mechanism whose transducers are represented by the sensitive endings of afferent sympathetic fibers widely distributed in the heart and vessels. The stimulation of these afferents increases, rather than reducing, the *error signal* and thus does not have a compensatory action, hence the sign *plus,* connoting the *positive feedback* mechanism. Such a mechanism has often been considered as a biological absurdity and probably it would be so if it were not only part of a complex regulatory system possessed, in stable conditions, of prevalent *negative feedback* properties. The interaction of opposite mechanisms, however, may better regulate the baseline and the range and velocity of changes affecting the regulated variable.

A similar schema (Figure 16) is applied to the neural regulation of sympathovagal balance. Also in this case baroreceptive and vagal afferent fibers from the cardiopulmonary region mediate *negative feedback* mechanisms (exciting the vagal outflow and inhibiting the sympathetic outflow), whereas *positive feedback* mechanisms are mediated by sympathetic afferent fibers (exciting the sympathetic outflow and inhibiting the vagal outflow).

Cardiovascular innervation schema

In the traditional conception of cardiovascular neural regulation, afferent fibers projecting from the cardiovascular system to

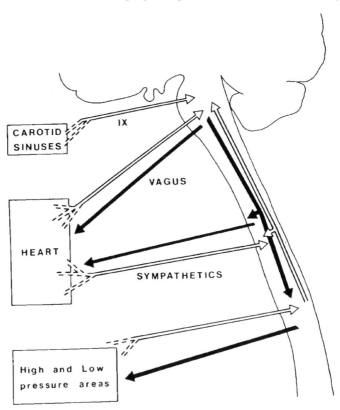

Figure 55: See text. (From Malliani 1982, with permission).

the supraspinal centers, and in particular to the medulla, were the only ones considered to originate from cardiovascular reflexogenic areas.In the schema of Figure 55, these afferent fibers include baroreceptive afferents originating from the carotid sinuses and running in the IX pair of cranial nerves and the cardiac vagal afferents.

Obviously, other important contingents of afferent fibers projecting to the medulla exist, although not represented in this schema: it is the case of chemoreceptive afferents from the carotid and aortic bodies and baroreceptive afferents from the aorta.

However the schema also includes the cardiovascular sympathetic innervation, conceived as an input-output system interacting with supraspinal mechanisms. As analyzed in *Chapter 1,* the sympathetic nervous system was considered in the traditional view as a pure outflow and, accordingly, the regulation of its activity was exclusively attributed to supraspinal centers. On the other hand, the now soundly proved reflexogenic role of cardiovascular sympathetic afferent fibers stresses the importance of defining, in addition to their functional properties, their course from an anatomical point of view (Malliani 1982).

Cardiovascular sympathetic afferent fibers have their receptor endings in the cardiovascular system, run through the sympathetic nerves and through the rami communicantes to reach the dorsal ganglia of spinal nerves, where their cell bodies are located, and therefrom impinge upon the spinal cord through the dorsal roots. Hence their afferent impulse activity can be unequivocally recorded from the cut peripheral end of the rami communicantes. Conversely, cardiac nerves include both vagal and sympathetic afferent and efferent fibers, a notion necessary to interpret numerous experimental findings.

Reflexes mediated by cardiovascular sympathetic afferents can be abolished by interrupting this afferent pathway – a procedure that can be performed at various anatomical sites, the most selective approach being however represented by sectioning the thoracic dorsal roots.

REFERENCES

Abraham F, Bryant H, Mettler M, Bergerson B, Moore F, Maderdrut J, Gardiner M, Walter D, Jennrich R (1973) Spectrum and discriminant analyses reveal remote rather than local sources for hypothalamic EEG: could waves affect unit activity? Brain Res 49:349-366.

Adgey AAJ, Geddes JS, Mulholland HC, Keegan DAJ, Pantridge JF (1968) Incidence, significance and management of early bradyarrhythmia complicating acute myocardial infarction. Lancet 2:1097-1101.

Adrian ED, Bronk DW, Phillips G (1932) Discharges in mammalian sympathetic nerves. J Physiol (Lond) 74:115-133.

Ajiki K, Murakawa Y, Yanagisawa-Miwa A, Usui M, Yamashita T, Oikawa N, Inoue H (1993) Autonomic nervous system activity in idiopathic dilated cardiomyopathy and in hypertrophic cardiomyopathy. Am J Cardiol 71:1316-1320.

Akselrod S, Gordon D, Ubel FA, Shannon DC, Barger AC, Cohen RJ (1981) Power spectrum analysis of heart rate fluctuation: a quantitative probe of beat-to-beat cardiovascular control. Science 213:220-222.

Akselrod S, Gordon D, Madwed JB, Snidman NC, Shannon DC, Cohen RJ (1985) Hemodynamic regulation: investigation by spectral analysis. Am J Physiol 249:H867-H875.

Akselrod S, Oz O, Greenberg M, Keselbrener L (1997) Autonomic response to change of posture among normal and mild-hypertensive adults: investigation by time-dependent spectral analysis. J Autonom Nerv Syst 64:33-43.

Alexander RS (1945) The effects of blood flow and anoxia on spinal cardiovascular centers. Am J Physiol 143:698-708.

Ammons SN, Blair RW, Hindorf K, Foreman RD (1983) Vagal afferent inhibition of spinothalamic cell responses to sympathetic afferents and bradykinin in the monkey. Circ Res 53:603-612.

Anderson EA, Sinkey CA, Lawton WJ, Mark AL (1989) Elevated sympathetic nerve activity in borderline hypertensive humans: evidence from direct intraneural recordings. Hypertension 14:177-183.

Ando S, Dajani HR, Senn BL, Newton GE, Floras JS (1997) Sympathetic alternans. Evidence for arterial baroreflex control of muscle sympathetic nerve activity in congestive heart failure. Circulation 95:316-319.

Anonymous (1988) Ying and Yang in vasomotor control. Lancet 2:19-20.

Appel ML, Berger RD, Saul JP, Smith JM, Cohen RJ (1989) Beat to beat variability in cardiovascular variables: noise or music? J Am Coll Cardiol 14:1139-48.

Atchley DW (1967) Patient-physician communication. In: Cecil-Loeb Textbook of Medicine, 12th edition, W.B. Saunders Co., Philadelphia, pp. 1-2.

Bainbridge FA (1915) The influence of venous filling upon the rate of the heart. J Physiol (Lond) 50:65-84.

Baker DG, Coleridge HM, Coleridge JCG, Nerdrum T (1980) Search for a cardiac nociceptor: stimulation by bradykinin of sympathetic afferent nerve endings in the heart of the cat. J Physiol (Lond) 306:519-536.

Bannister R (1979) Chronic autonomic failure with postural hypotension. Lancet 2:404-406.

Barber MJ, Mueller M, Davies BG, Zipes DP (1984) Phenol topically applied to canine left ventricular epicardium interrupts sympathetic but not vagal afferents. Circ Res 55:532-544.

Bard P (1928) A diencephalic mechanism for the expression of rage with special reference to the sympathetic nervous system. Am J Physiol 84: 490-515.

Bard P (1960) Anatomical organization of the central nervous system in relation to control of the heart and blood vessels. Physiol Rev (suppl) 40: 3-26.

Barnett SR, Morin RJ, Kiely DK, Gagnon M, Azhar G, Knight EL, Nelson JC, Lipsitz LA (1999) Effects of age and gender on autonomic control of blood pressure dynamics. Circulation 33:1195-1200.

Barron KW, Bishop VS (1982) Reflex cardiovascular changes with veratridine in the conscious dog. Am J Physiol 242:H810-H817.

Barsky AJ (1986) Palliation and symptomatic relief. Arch Intern Med 146: 905-909.

Bartorelli C, Bizzi E, Libretti A, Zanchetti A (1960) Inhibitory control of sinocarotid pressoceptive afferents on hypothalamic autonomic activity and sham rage behavior. Arch Ital Biol 98, 308-326.

Baselli G, Cerutti S, Civardi S, Lombardi F, Malliani A, Pagani M (1986) Methodological aspects for studying the relations between heart rate and blood pressure variability signals. In: Lown B, Malliani A, Prosdocimi M (eds), Neural mechanisms and cardiovascular disease. Liviana Press, Springer Verlag. Padova, Berlin, pp 251-264.

Baselli G, Cerutti S, Civardi S, Malliani A, Pagani M (1988) Cardiovascular variability signals. Towards the identification of a closed-loop model of the neural control mechanisms. IEEE Trans Biomed Eng 35:1033-1046.

Beacham WS, Kunze DL (1969) Renal receptors evoking a spinal vasomotor reflex. J Physiol (Lond) 201:73-85.

Beacham WS, Perl ER (1964) Background and reflex discharge of sympathetic preganglionic neurones in the spinal cat. J Physiol (Lond) 172:400-416.

Bellavere F, Balzani I, De Masi G, Carraro M, Carenza P, Cobelli C, Thomaseth K (1992) Power spectral analysis of heart-rate variations improves assessment of diabetic cardiac autonomic neuropathy. Diabetes 41:633-640.

Bergamaschi M (1978) Role of sympathetic and parasympathetic innervation in the genesis of ventricular arrhythmias during experimental myocardial ischemia. In: Schwartz PJ, Brown AM, Malliani A, Zanchetti A (eds.), Neural mechanisms in cardiac arrhythmias. Raven Press, New York pp 139-154.

Bergamaschi M, Longoni AM (1973) Cardiovascular events in anxiety: experimental studies in the conscious dog. Am Heart J 86: 385-394.

Bernard C (1876) Leçons sur la chaleur animale. J-B Baillière et fils, Paris.

Bernard C (1878) Leçons sur les phénomènes de la vie communs aux animaux et aux végétaux. J-B Baillière et fils, Paris.

Bernardi L, Keller F, Sanders M, Reddy PS, Griffith B, Meno F, Pinsky MR (1989) Respiratory sinus arrhythmia in the denervated human heart. J Appl Physiol 67:1447-1455.

Bernardi L, Ricordi L, Lazzari P, Soldà P, Calciati A, Ferrari MR, Vandea I, Finardi G, Fratino P (1992) Impaired circadian modulation of sympathovagal activity in diabetes. A possible explanation for altered temporal onset of cardiovascular disease. Circulation 86:1443-1452.

Bernardi L, Valle F, Coco M, Calciati A, Sleight P (1996) Physical activity influences heart rate variability and very-low-frequency components in Holter electrocardiograms. Cardiovasc Res 32:234-237.

Bernardi L, Passino C, Robergs R, Appenzeller O (1997) Acute and persistent effects of a 46-kilometre wilderness trail run at altitude: cardiovascular autonomic modulation and baroreflexes. Cardiovasc Res 34:273-280.

Bernardi L, Valenti C, Wdowczyck-Szulc J, Frey AW, Rinaldi M, Spadacini G, Passino C, Martinelli L, Viganò M, Finardi G (1998) Influence of type of surgery on the occurrence of parasympathetic reinnervation after cardiac transplantation. Circulation 97:1368-1374.

Bertinieri G, Di Rienzo M, Cavallazzi A, Ferrari AU, Pedotti A, Mancia G (1988) Evaluation of baroreceptor reflex by blood pressure monitoring in unanesthetized cats. Am J Physiol 254:H377-H383.

Biagini A, Emdin M, Michelassi C, Mazzei C, Carpeggiani C, Testa R, Andreotti F, L'Abbate A (1988) The contribution of ventricular tachyarrhythmias to the genesis of cardiac pain during transient myocardial ischemia in patients with variant angina. Eur Heart J 6:182-188.

Bianchi A, Mainardi L, Signorini MG, Cerutti S, Lombardi F, Montefusco A, Malliani A (1992) Time-variant spectral estimation of heart rate variability signal. Comput Cardiol 265-268.

Bigger JT, Kleiger RE, Fleiss JL, Rolnitzky LM, Steinman RC, Miller JP, Multicenter post-infarction research group (1988) Components of heart rate variability measured during healing of acute myocardial infarction. Am J Cardiol 61:208-215.

Bigger JT, Fleiss JL, Steinman RC, Rolnitzky LM, Kleiger RE, Rottman JN (1992) Frequency domain measures of heart period variability and mortality after myocardial infarction. Circulation 85:164-171.

Bigger JT, Steinman RC, Rolnitzky LM, Fleiss JL, Albrecht P, Cohen RJ (1996) Power law behavior of RR-interval variability in healthy middle-aged persons, patients with recent acute myocardial infarction, and patients with heart transplants. Circulation 93:2142-2151.

Binkley PF, Nunziata E, Haas GJ, Nelson SD, Cody RJ (1991) Parasympathetic withdrawal is an integral component of autonomic imbalance in congestive heart failure: demonstration in human subjects and verification in a paced canine model of ventricular failure. J Am Coll Cardiol 18:464-472.

Bishop VS, Lombardi F, Malliani A, Pagani M, Recordati G (1976) Reflex sympathetic tachycardia during intravenous infusions in chronic spinal cats. Am J Physiol 230:25-29.

Bishop VS, Malliani A, Thorén P (1983) Cardiac mechanoreceptors. In: Shepherd JT, Abboud FM, Geiger SR (eds) Handbook of physiology. Section 2. The Cardiovascular System, vol.III. Peripheral Circulation and Organ Blood Flow. American Physiological Society, Washington DC, pp.497-555.

Bizzi E, Libretti A, Malliani A, Zanchetti A (1961) Reflex chemoceptive excitation of diencephalic sham rage behavior. Am J Physiol 200:923-926.

Blaber AP, Bondar RL, Freeman R (1996) Coarse graining spectral analysis of HR and BP variability in patients with autonomic failure. Am J Physiol 271:H1555-H1564.

Blois MS (1988) Medicine and the nature of vertical reasoning. N Engl J Med 318:847-851.

Bodenheimer T (1999) The American health care system. The movement for improved quality in health care. N Engl J Med 340:488-492.

Bonaduce D, Petretta M, Piscione F, Indolfi C, Migaux ML, Bianchi V, Esposito N, Marciano F, Chiariello M (1994) Influence of reversible segmental left ventricular dysfunction on heart period variability in patients with one-vessel coronary artery disease. J Am Coll Cardiol 24:399-405.

Bootsma M, Swenne CA, Van Bolhuis HH, Chang PC, Manger Cats VM, Bruschke AVG (1994) Heart rate and heart rate variability as indexes of sympathovagal balance. Am J Physiol 266:H1565-H1571.

Bosnjak ZK, Zuperku EJ, Coon RL, Kampine JP (1979) Acute coronary artery occlusion and cardiac sympathetic afferent nerve activity. Proc Soc Exp Biol Med 161:142-148.

Bradbury S, Egglestone C (1925) Postural hypotension. A report of three cases. Am Heart J 1:73-86.

Brändle M, Patel KP, Wang W, Zucker IH (1996) Hemodynamic and norepinephrine responses to pacing-induced heart failure in conscious sinoaortic-denervated dogs. J Appl Physiol 81:1855-1862.

Bristow JD, Honour AJ, Pickering GW, Sleight P, Smyth HS (1969) Diminished baroreflex sensitivity in high blood pressure. Circulation 39:48-54.

Bristow JD, Brown EW, Cunningham DJC, Howson MG, Petersen ES, Pickering TG, Sleight P (1971) Effect of bicycling on the baroreflex regulation of pulse interval. Circ Res 28:582-592.

Bronk DW, Ferguson LK, Margaria R, Solandt DY (1936) The activity of the cardiac sympathetic centers. Am J Physiol 117:237-249.

Brooks CM (1933) Reflex activation of the sympathetic system in the spinal cat. Am J Physiol 106:251-266.

Brooks CM (1935) The reaction of chronic spinal animals to hemorrhage. Am J Physiol 114:30-39.

Brovelli M, Baselli G, Cerutti S, Guzzetti S, Liberati D, Lombardi F, Malliani A, Pagani M, Pizzinelli P (1983) Computerized analysis for an experimental validation of neurophysiological models of heart rate control. Comput Cardiol 205-208.

Brown AM (1967) Excitation of afferent cardiac sympathetic nerve fibres during myocardial ischaemia. J Physiol (Lond) 190:35-53.

Brown AM (1980) Receptors under pressure. Circ Res 46:1-10.

Brown AM, Malliani A (1971) Spinal sympathetic reflexes initiated by coronary receptors. J Physiol (Lond) 212:685-705.

Brown DR, Randall DC, Knapp CF, Lee KC, Yingling JD (1989) Stability of the heart rate power spectrum over time in the conscious dog. FASEB J 3:1644-1650.

Burgess PR, Perl ER (1973) Cutaneous mechanoreceptors and nociceptors. In: Iggo A (ed) Handbook of sensory physiology, vol 2. Somatosensory system. Springer, Berlin Heidelberg New York, pp. 29-78.

Cannon WB (1932) The wisdom of the body. W.W. Norton, New York.

Cannon WB (1945) The way of an investigator. Hafner Publishing Company, New York and London.

Cannon WB, Britton SW (1925) Studies on the conditions of activity in endocrine glands. XV. Pseudoaffective medulliadrenal secretion. Am J Physiol 72:283-294.

Carré F, Maison-Blanche P, Ollivier L, Mansier P, Chevalier B, Vicuna R, Lessard Y, Coumel P, Swynghedauw B (1994) Heart rate variability in two models of cardiac hypertrophy in rats in relation to the new molecular phenotype. Am J Physiol 266:H1872-H1878.

Casati R, Lombardi F, Malliani A (1979) Afferent sympathetic unmyelinated fibres with left ventricular endings in cats. J Physiol (Lond) 292:135-148.

Casolo G, Balli E, Taddei T, Amuhasi J, Gori C (1989) Decreased spontaneous heart rate variability in congestive heart failure. Am J Cardiol 64:1162-1167.

Cerutti S, Baselli G, Civardi S, Furlan R, Lombardi F, Malliani A, Merri M, Pagani M (1987) Spectral analysis of heart rate and arterial blood pressure variability signals for physiological and clinical purposes. Comput Cardiol 435-438.

Chakko S, Mulingtapang RF, Huikuri HV, Kessler KM, Materson BJ, Myerburg RJ (1993) Alterations in heart rate variability and its circadian rhythm in hypertensive patients with left ventricular hypertrophy free of coronary artery disease. Am Heart J 126:1364-1372.

Chess GF, Tam RMK, Calaresu FR (1975) Influence of cardiac neural inputs on rhythmic variations of heart period in the cat. Am J Physiol 228:775-780.

Chidsey CA, Harrison DC, Braunwald E (1962) Augmentation of plasma norepinephrine response to exercise in patients with congestive heart failure. N Engl J Med 267:650-654.

Chierchia S, Muiesan L, Davies A, Balasubramian V, Gerosa S, Raftery EB. (1990) Role of the sympathetic nervous system in the pathogenesis of chronic stable angina. Circulation 82(suppl): II-71 - II-81.

Cohn JN, Levine TB, Olivari MT, Garberg V, Lura D, Francis GS, Simon AB, Rector T (1984) Plasma norepinephrine as a guide to prognosis in patients with chronic congestive heart failure. N Engl J Med 311:819-823.

Cohn PF (1980) Silent myocardial ischemia in patients with a defective anginal warning system. Am J Cardiol 45: 697-702.

Colbeck EH (1903) Angina pectoris: a criticism and a hypothesis. Lancet i:793-795.

Coleridge HM, Kidd C, Coleridge JCG, Banzett RB (1975) Multiterminal sympathetic afferent fibers supplying the thoracic organs of cats and dogs. Physiologist 18:173.

Coleridge JCG, Coleridge HM (1979) Chemoreflex regulation of the heart. In: Berne RM, Sperelakis N, Geiger SR (eds) Handbook of physiology. 2. The cardiovascular system, vol. I The heart. American Physiological Society, Washington DC, pp 653-676.

Comte A (1828) Examen du traité de Broussais sur l'irritation. In: Comte A: Ecrits de Jeunesse (1816-1828). Monton, Paris, 1970.

Consensus Committee of the American Autonomic Society and the American Academy of Neurology (1996) Consensus statement on the definition of orthostatic hypotension, pure autonomic failure, and multiple system atrophy. J Neurol Sci 144:218-219.

Cooke WH, Hoag JB, Crossman AA, Kuusela TA, Tahvanainen KUO, Eckberg DL (1999) Human responses to upright tilt: a window on central autonomic integration. J Physiol (Lond) 517.2:617-628.

Cooley JW, Tukey JW (1965) An algorithm for the machine calculation of complex Fourier Series. Math Comput 19:289-301.

Cooley RL, Montano N, Cogliati C, van de Borne P, Richenbacher W, Oren R, Somers VK (1998) Evidence for a central origin of the low-frequency oscillation in RR interval variability. Circulation. 98:556-561.

Coote JH, Hilton SM, Perez-Gonzales JF (1971) The reflex nature of the pressor response to muscular exercise. J Physiol (Lond) 215: 789-804.

Corbett JL, Frankel HL, Harris PJ (1971a) Cardiovascular changes associated with skeletal muscle spasm in tetraplegic man. J Physiol (Lond) 215:381-393.

Corbett JL, Frankel HL, Harris PJ (1971b) Cardiovascular reflex responses to cutaneous and visceral stimuli in spinal man. J Physiol (Lond) 215:395-409.

Corr PB and Gillis RA (1974) Role of the vagus nerves in the cardiovascular changes induced by coronary occlusion. Circulation 49:86-97.

Costantin LR (1963) Extracardiac factors contributing to hypotension during coronary occlusion. Am J Cardiol 11:205-217.

Coumel P (1990) Noninvasive exploration of cardiac arrhythmias. Ann NY Acad Sci 601:312-328.

Cowley AW, Guyton AC (1975) Baroreceptor reflex effects on transient and steady-state hemodynamics of salt-loading hypertension in dogs. Circ Res 36:536-546.

Crea F, Pupita G, Galassi AR, El-Tamini H, Kaski JC, Davies G, Maseri A (1990) Role of adenosine in pathogenesis of anginal pain. Circulation 81:893-904.

Cyon E, Ludwig C (1866) Die Reflexe eines der sensiblen Nerven des Herzens auf die motorischen der Blutgefässe. Ber Saechs Ges (Akad) Wiss 18:307-328.

Dalla Vecchia L, Mangini A, Di Biasi P, Santoli C, Malliani A (1998) Improvement of left ventricular function and cardiovascular neural control after endoventriculoplasty and myocardial revascularization. Cardiovasc Res 37:101-107.

Daly RN, Hieble JP. (1987) Neuropeptide Y modulates adrenergic neurotransmission by an endothelium dependent mechanism. Eur J Pharmacol 138:445-46.

Darwin E (1794) Zoönomia, or the laws of organic life. J Johnson, London, vol 1.

DeBoer RW (1985) Beat-to-beat blood-pressure fluctuations and heart-rate variability in man: Physiological relationships, analysis techniques and a simple model. Amsterdam, University of Amsterdam. Thesis.

DeBoer RW, Karemaker JM, van Montfrans GA (1986) Determination of baroreflex sensitivity by spectral analysis of spontaneous blood-pressure and heart-rate fluctuations in man. In: Lown B, Malliani A, Prosdocimi M (eds), Neural mechanisms and cardiovascular disease. Liviana Press, Springer Verlag. Padova, Berlin, pp 303-315.

De Ferrari GM, Vanoli E, Schwartz PJ (1994) Vagal activity and ventricular fibrillation. In Levy MN, Schwartz PJ (eds.), Vagal control of the heart: experimental basis and clinical implications. Futura Publishing Co. Inc., Armonk, NY, pp 613-636.

Denton TA, Diamond GA, Helfant RH, Khan S, Karagueuzian H (1990) Fascinating rhythm: A primer on chaos theory and its application to cardiology. Am Heart J 120:1419-1440.

De Waele H, Van de Velde J (1940) Sur un réflexe hypertenseur des oreillettes. Arch Int Physiol 50:33-53.

Dickinson CJ (1993) Fainting precipitated by collapse-firing of venous baroreceptors. Lancet 342:970-972.

Downmann CBB, McSwiney BA (1946) Reflexes elicited by visceral stimulation in the acute spinal animal. J Physiol (Lond) 105:80-94.

Droste C, Greenlee MW, Roskamm H (1986) A defective angina pectoris pain warning system: experimental findings of ischemic and electrical pain test. Pain 26: 199-209.

Eaton GM, Cody RJ, Nunziata E, Binkley PF (1995) Early left ventricular dysfunction elicits activation of sympathetic drive and attenuation of parasympathetic tone in the paced canine model of congestive heart failure. Circulation 92:555-561.

Eckberg DL (1997) Sympathovagal balance: a critical appraisal. Circulation 96:3224-3232.

Eckberg DL, Drabinsky M, Braunwald E (1971) Defective cardiac parasympathetic control in patients with heart disease. N Engl J Med 285:877-883.

Eckmann JP, Kamphorst OS, Ruelle D, Ciliberto S (1986) Lyapunov exponents from time series. Phys Rev A 34:4971-4979.

Edgeworth FH (1892) On a large-fibred sensory supply of the thoracic and abdominal viscera. J Physiol (Lond) 13:260-271.

Eisenhofer G, Friberg P, Rundqvist B, Quyyumi AA, Lambert G, Kaye DM, Kopin IJ, Goldstein DS, Esler MD (1996) Cardiac sympathetic nerve function in congestive heart failure. Circulation 93:1667-1676.

Esler M, Lambert G, Jennings G (1990) Increased regional sympathetic nervous activity in human hypertension: causes and consequences. J Hyperten 8:S53-S57.

Ewing DJ, Campbell IW, Clarke BF (1976) Mortality in diabetic autonomic neuropathy. Lancet 1:601-603.

Ewing DJ, Martyn CN, Young RJ, Clarke BF (1985) The value of cardiovascular autonomic function tests: 10 years experience in diabetes. Diabetes Care 8:491-498.

Fagard RH, Pardaens K, Staessen JA, Thijs L (1998) Power spectral analysis of heart rate variability by autoregressive modelling and fast Fourier transform: a comparative study. Acta Cardiol 53:211-218.

Fagard RH, Pardaens K, Staessen JA (1999) Influence of demographic, anthropometric and lifestyle characteristics on heart rate and its variability in the population. J Hypertens 17:1589-1599.

Fallen EL, Kamath MV, Ghista DN, Fitchett D (1988) Spectral analysis of heart rate variability following human heart transplantation: Evidence for functional reinnervation. J Autonom Nerv Syst 23:199-206.

Farrel TG, Bashir Y, Cripps TR, Malik M, Poloniecki J, Bennet ED, Ward DE, Camm AJ (1991) Risk stratification for arrhythmic events in post-infarction patients based on heart rate variability, ambulatory electrocardiogram. J Am Coll Cardiol 18:687-697.

Feigl EO (1983) Coronary physiology. Physiol Rev 63:1-205.

Felder RB, Thames MD (1979) Interaction between cardiac receptors and sinoaortic baroreceptors in the control of efferent cardiac sympathetic nerve activity during myocardial ischemia in dogs. Circ Res 45:728-736.

Ferguson DW, Berg WJ, Roach PJ, Oren RM, Mark AL, Kempf JS (1992) Effects of heart failure on baroreflex control of sympathetic neural activity. Am J Cardiol 69:523-531.

Fernandez de Molina A, Perl ER (1965) Sympathetic activity and the systemic circulation in the spinal cat. J Physiol (Lond) 181:82-102.

Ferrannini E, Buzzigoli G, Bonadonna R, Giorico MA, Oleggini M, Graziadei L, Pedrinelli R, Brandi L, Bevilacqua S (1987) Insulin resistance in essential hypertension. N Engl J Med 317:350-357.

Feyerabend PK (1975) Against method. Verso, London.

Folkow B (1982) Physiological aspects of primary hypertension. Physiol Rev 62:347-504.

Foreman RD (1986) Spinothalamic tract and cardiac afferents. In: Lown B, Malliani A, Prosdocimi P (eds) Fidia research series. Liviana Press, Padova, Springer, Berlin Heidelberg New York, pp. 169-181.

Foreman RD, Ohata CA (1980) Effects of coronary artery occlusion on thoracic spinal neurons receiving viscerosomatic inputs. Am J Physiol 238: H667-H674.

Fouad FM, Tadena-Thome L, Bravo EL, Tarazi RC (1986) Idiopathic hypovolemia. Arch Intern Med 104:298-303.

Franz DN, Evans MH, Perl ER (1966) Characteristics of viscerosympathetic reflexes in the spinal cat. Am J Physiol 211:1292-1298.

Furberg CD, Psaty BM, Meyer JV (1995) Nifedipine. Dose-related increase in mortality in patients with coronary heart disease. Circulation 92:1326-1331.

Furchgott RF, Zawadzki JV (1980) The obligatory role of endothelial cells in the relaxation of arterial smooth muscle by acetylcholine. Nature 288:373-376.

Furlan R, Dell'Orto S, Crivellaro W, Pizzinelli P, Cerutti S, Lombardi F, Pagani M, Malliani A (1987) Effects of tilt and treadmill exercise on short-term variability in systolic arterial pressure in hypertensive men. J Hypertens 5(suppl 5):S423-S425.

Furlan R, Guzzetti S, Crivellaro W, Dassi S, Tinelli M, Baselli G, Cerutti S, Lombardi F, Pagani M, Malliani A (1990) Continuous 24-hour assessment of the neural regulation of systemic arterial pressure and RR variabilities in ambulant subjects. Circulation 81:537-547

Furlan R, Gentile E, Piazza S, Dell'Orto S, Barbic F, Pagani MR, Lombardi F, Pagani M, Malliani A (1991) Increased vascular sympathetic activity at rest and reduced responsiveness to excitatory stimuli in essential hypertension. J Hypertens 9 (suppl 6):S60-S61.

Furlan R, Piazza S, Dell'Orto S, Gentile E, Cerutti S, Pagani M, Malliani A (1993) Early and late effects of exercise and athletic training on neural mechanisms controlling heart rate. Cardiovasc Res 27:482-488.

Furlan R, Piazza S, Bevilacqua M, Turiel M, Norbiato G, Lombardi F, Malliani A (1995) Pure autonomic failure: complex abnormalities in the neural mechanisms regulating the cardiovascular system. J Autonom Nerv Syst 51:223-235.

Furlan R, Jacob G, Snell M, Robertson D, Porta A, Harris P, Mosqueda-Garcia R (1998a) Chronic orthostatic intolerance. A disorder with discordant cardiac and vascular sympathetic control. Circulation 98:2154-2159.

Furlan R, Piazza S, Dell'Orto S, Barbic F, Bianchi A, Mainardi L, Cerutti S, Pagani M, Malliani A (1998b) Cardiac autonomic patterns preceding occasional vasovagal reactions in healthy humans. Circulation 98:1756-1761.

Furlan R, Porta A, Costa F, Tank J, Baker L, Schiavi R, Robertson D, Malliani A, Mosqueda-Garcia R (2000) Oscillatory patterns in sympathetic neural discharge and cardiovascular variables during orthostatic stimulus. Circulation (in press).

Garrard CS, Seidler A, McKibben A, McAlpine LE, Gordon D (1992) Spectral analysis of heart rate variability in bronchial asthma. Clin Autonom Res 2:105-111.

Gerstner W, Kreiter AK, Markram H, Herz AVM (1997) Neural codes: Firing rates and beyond. Proc Natl Acad Sci 94:12740-12741.

Glass L, Mackey MC (1998) From clock to chaos: the rhythms of life. Princeton University Press, Princeton.

Gnecchi Ruscone T, Lombardi F, Malfatto G, Malliani A (1987) Attenuation of baroreceptive mechanisms by cardiovascular sympathetic afferent fibers. Am J Physiol 253:H787-H791.

Gnecchi Ruscone T, Montano N, Contini M, Guazzi M, Lombardi F, Malliani A (1995) Adenosine activates cardiac sympathetic afferent fibers and potentiates the excitation induced by coronary occlusion. J Autonom Nerv Syst 53:175-184.

Goldberger AL, West BJ (1987) Applications of non linear dynamics to clinical cardiology. Ann NY Acad Sci 504:195-213.

Goldberger JJ (1999) Sympathetic balance: how should we measure it? Am J Physiol 276:H1273-H1280.

Goldsmith RL, Bigger JT Jr, Steinman RC, Fleiss JL (1992) Comparison of 24-hour parasympathetic activity in endurance-trained and untrained young men. J Am Coll Cardiol 20:552-558.

Goldstein DS (1981) Plasma norepinephrine in essential hypertension: a study of the studies. Hypertension 27:520-529.

Gooddy W (1957) On the nature of pain. Brain 80: 118-131.

Gottlieb SS, McCarter RJ, Vogel RA (1998) Effect of beta-blockade on mortality among high-risk and low-risk patients after myocardial infarction. N Engl J Med 339:489-497.

Grassberger P, Procaccia I (1983) Measuring the strangeness of strange attractors. Physica D 9: 189-208.

Grassi G, Esler M (1999) How to assess sympathetic activity in humans. J Hypertens 17:719-734.

Greenwood JP, Stoker JB, Mary DASG (1999) Single-unit sympathetic discharge. Quantitative assessment in human hypertensive disease. Circulation 100:1305-1310.

Gregorini L, Fajadet J, Robert G, Cassagneau B, Bernis M, Marco J (1994) Coronary vasoconstriction following percutaneous transluminal coronary angioplasty is attenuated by antiadrenergic agents. Circulation 90:895-907.

Griffith TM (1996) Temporal chaos in the microcirculation. Cardiovasc Res 31:342-358.

Grimm DR, De Meersman RE, Almenoff PL, Spungen AM, Bauman WA (1997) Sympathovagal balance of the heart in subjects with spinal cord injury. Am J Physiol 272:H835-H842.

Guazzi M, Polese A, Fiorentini C, Magrini F, Bartorelli C (1971) Left ventricular performance and related haemodynamic changes in Prinzmetal's variant angina pectoris. Br Heart J 33:84-94.

Guazzi M, Polese A, Fiorentini C, Magrini F, Olivari MT, Bartorelli C (1975) Left and right heart haemodynamics during spontaneous angina pectoris. Comparison between angina with ST segment depression and angina with ST segment elevation. Br Heart J 37:401-413.

Guevara MR Shrier A, Glass L (1988) Phase-locked rhythms in periodically stimulated heart cell aggregates. Am J Physiol 254:H1-H10.

Gupta PD (1975) Spinal autonomic afferents in elicitation of tachycardia in volume infusion in the dog. Am J Physiol 229:303-308.

Gupta PD, Singh M (1977) Autonomic afferents at T1 in elicitation of volume-induced tachycardia in the dog. Am J Physiol 232:H464-H469.

Guttman F, Whitteridge D (1947) Effects of bladder distension on autonomic mechanisms after spinal cord injuries. Brain 70:361-404.

Guyton AC, Coleman TG, Cowley AW Jr., Manning RD Jr., Norman RA Jr., Ferguson JD (1974) A systems analysis approach to understanding long-range arterial blood pressure control and hypertension. Circ Res 35:159-176.

Guzman F, Braun C, Lim RKS (1962) Visceral pain and the pseudoaffective response to intra-arterial injection of bradykinin and other algesic agents. Arch Intern Pharmacodyn Ther 136: 353-384.

Guzzetti S, Piccaluga E, Casati R, Cerutti S, Lombardi F, Pagani M, Malliani A (1988) Sympathetic predominance in essential hypertension: a study employing spectral analysis of heart rate variability. J Hypertens 6:711-717.

Guzzetti S, Dassi S, Pecis M, Casati R, Masu AM, Longoni P, Tinelli M, Cerutti S, Pagani M, Malliani A (1991a) Altered pattern of circadian neural control of heart period in mild hypertension. J Hypertens 9:831-838.

Guzzetti S, Iosa D, Pecis M, Bonura L, Prosdocimi M, Malliani A (1991b) Impaired heart rate variability in patients with chronic Chagas' disease. Am Heart J 121:1727-1734.

Guzzetti S, Cogliati C, Broggi C, Carozzi C, Caldiroli D, Lombardi F, Malliani A (1994a) Influences of neural mechanisms on heart period and arterial pressure variabilities in quadriplegic patients. Am J Physiol 266:H1112-H1120.

Guzzetti S, Dassi S, Balsamà M, Ponti GB, Pagani M, Malliani A (1994b) Altered dynamics of the circadian relationship between systemic arterial pressure and cardiac sympathetic drive early on in mild hypertension. Clin Sci 86:209-215.

Guzzetti S, Cogliati C, Turiel M, Crema C, Lombardi F, Malliani A (1995) Sympathetic predominance followed by functional denervation in the progression of chronic heart failure. Europ Heart J 16:1100-1107.

Guzzetti S, Signorini MG, Cogliati C, Mezzetti S, Porta A, Cerutti S, Malliani A (1996) Non-linear dynamics and chaotic indices in heart rate variability of normal subjects and heart-transplanted patients. Cardiovasc Res 31:441-446.

Hales S (1733) Statical essays: containing haemastaticks. Innys, Manby and Woodward. London, England. (Volume 2).

Handwerker HO (1984) Experimentelle Schmerzanalyse beim Menschen. In: Zimmermann M, Handewerker HO (eds) Schmerz, Springer, Berlin Heidelberg New York, pp 87-123.

Hayano J, Sakakibara Y, Yamada M, Ohte N, Fujinami T, Yokoyama K, Watanabe Y, Takata K (1990) Decreased magnitude of heart rate spectral components in coronary artery disease. 81:1217-1224.

Head H (1921) Release of function in the nervous system. Proc Roy Soc Lond (Biol) 92:184-209.

Hedman AE, Tahvanainen KUO, Hartikainen JEK, Hakumäki MOK (1995) Effect of sympathetic modulation and sympatho-vagal interaction on heart rate variability in anaesthetized dogs. Acta Physiol Scand 155:205-214.

Heller A (1974) La teoria dei bisogni in Marx. Feltrinelli Editore, Milano.

Henry JP, Stephens PM, Santisteban GA (1975) A model of psychosocial hypertension showing reversibility and progression of cardiovascular complications. Circ Res 36:156-164.

Henry JP, Liu YY, Nadra WE, Qian CG, Mormede P, Lemaire V, Ely D, Hendley ED (1993) Psychosocial stress can induce chronic hypertension in normotensive strains of rats. Hypertension 21:714-723.

Herd JA, Morse WH, Kelleher RT, Jones LG (1969) Arterial hypertension in the squirrel monkey during behavioral experiments. Am J Physiol 217:24-29.

Herman J (1998) The good old days. Lancet 352:1930-1931.

Hess GL, Zuperku EJ, Coon RL, Kampine JP (1974) Sympathetic afferent nerve activity of left ventricular origin. Am J Physiol 227:543-546.

Hess WR (1957) The functional organization of the diencephalon. New York, New York: Grune & Stratton Inc., 1957.

Heusch G, Deussen A, Thamer V (1985) Cardiac sympathetic nerve activity and progressive vasoconstriction distal to coronary stenoses: feedback aggravation of myocardial ischemia. J Auton Nerv Syst 13:311-326.

Heymans C (1929) Le sinus carotidien. H. K. Lewis, London.

Heymans C, Neil E (1958) Reflexogenic areas of the cardiovascular system. Churchill, London.

Heymans C, Bouckaert JJ, Farber S, Hsu FY (1936) Spinal vasomotor reflexes associated with variations in blood pressure. Am J Physiol 117:619-625.

Hickey KA, Rubanyr GM, Paul RJ, Highsmith RF (1985) Characterization of a coronary vasoconstrictor produced by cultured endothelial cells. Am J Physiol 248:C550-56.

Higgins CB, Vatner SF, Eckberg DL, Braunwald E (1972) Alterations in the baroreceptor reflex in conscious dogs with congestive heart failure. J Clin Invest 51:715-724.

Hilton SM (1966) Hypothalamic regulation of the cardiovascular system. Br Med Bull 22:243-248.

Hoffman BB, Lefkowitz JR (1996) Catecholamines, sympathomimetic drugs, and adrenergic receptor antagonist. In: Hardman JG, Limbird LE (eds) Goodman and Gilman's The Pharmacological Basis of Therapeutics, 9th edn. McGraw-Hill, New York, pp 199-249.

Houk J, Henneman E (1974) Feedback control of muscle: introductory concepts. In: Mountcastle VB (ed.), Medical Physiology 13th edn., Mosby Co., Saint Louis, pp. 608-616.

Horton R (1999) The use of error. Lancet 353:422-423.

Hyndman BW, Kitney RI, Sayers BM (1971) Spontaneous rhythms in physiological control systems. Nature 233:339-341.

Huikuri HV, Linnaluoto MK, Seppänen T, Airaksinen KEJ, Kessler KM, Takkunen JT, Myerburg RJ (1992) Heart rate variability and its circadian rhythm in survivors of cardiac arrest. Am J Cardiol 70:610-615.

Huikuri HV, Valkama JO, Airaksinen KEJ, Seppänen T, Kessler KM, Takkunen JT, Myerburg RJ (1993) Frequency domain measures of heart rate variability before the onset of nonsustained and sustained ventricular tachycardia in patients with coronary artery disease. Circulation 87:1220-1228.

Huikuri HV, Pikkujämsä SM, Airaksinen KEJ, Ikäheimo MJ, Rantala AO, Kauma H, Lilja M, Kesaniemi A (1996a) Sex-related differences in autonomic modulation of heart rate in middle-aged subjects. Circulation 94:122-125.

Huikuri HV, Ylitalo A, Pikkujämsä SM, Ikäheimo MJ, Airaksinen KEJ, Rantala AO, Lilja M, Kesäniemi YA (1996b) Heart rate variability in systemic hypertension. Am J Cardiol 77:1073-1077.

Ibrahim MM, Tarazi RC, Dustan HP, Bravo EL (1974) Idiopathic orthostatic hypotension: circulatory dynamics in chronic autonomic insufficiency. Am J Cardiol 34:288-294.

Iellamo F, Pizzinelli P, Massaro M, Raimondi G, Peruzzi G, Legramante JM (1999) Muscle metaboreflex contribution to sinus node regulation during static exercise. Insights from spectral analysis of heart rate variability. Circulation 100:27-32.

Ignarro LJ, Buga GM, Wood KS, Byrns RE, Chaudhuri G (1987) Endothelium-derived relaxing factor produced and released from artery and vein is nitric oxide. Proc Natl Acad Sci USA. 84:9265-9269.

Illich I (1975) Medical nemesis. Marion Boyars, London.

Inoue K, Miyake S, Kumashiro M, Ogata H, Yoshimura O (1990) Power spectral analysis of heart rate variability in traumatic quadriplegic humans. Am J Physiol 258:H1722-H1726.

Inoue K, Miyake S, Kumashiro M, Ogata H, Ueta T, Akatsu T (1991) Power spectral analysis of blood pressure variability in traumatic quadriplegic humans. Am J Physiol 260:H842-H847.

Introna R, Yodlowski E, Pruett J, Montano N, Porta A, Crumrine R (1995) Sympathovagal effects of spinal anesthesia assessed by heart rate variability analysis. Anesth Analg 80:315-321.

Ishise H, Asanoi H, Ishizaka S, Joho S, Kameyama T, Umeno K, Inoue H (1998) Time course of sympathovagal imbalance and left ventricular dysfunction in conscious dogs with heart failure. J Appl Physiol 84:1234-1241.

Japundzic N, Grichois ML, Zitoun P, Laude D, Elghozi JL (1990) Spectral analysis of blood pressure and heart rate in conscious rats: effects of autonomic blockers. J Autonom Nerv Syst 30:91-100.

Jasson S, Médigue C, Maison-Blanche P, Montano N, Meyer L, Vermeiren C, Mansier P, Coumel P, Malliani A, Swynghedauw B (1997) Instant power spectrum analysis of heart rate variability during orthostatic tilt using a time-/frequency-domain method. Circulation 96:3521-3526.

Jewett DL (1964) Activity of single efferent fibres in the cervical vagus nerve of the dog, with special reference to possible cardio-inhibitory fibres. J Physiol (Lond) 175:321-357.

Jonnesco T (1921) Traitement chirurgical de l'angine de poitrine par la résection du sympathique cervico-thoracique. Press Méd 29: 193-194.

Julius S (1991) Autonomic nervous system dysregulation in human hypertension. Am J Cardiol 67:3B-7B.

Kagiyama S, Tsukashima A, Abe I, Fujishima S, Ohmori S, Onaka U Ohya Y, Fujii K, Tsuchihashi T, Fujishima M (1999) Chaos and spectral analyses of heart rate variability during head-up tilting in essential hypertension. J Autonom Nerv Syst 76:153-158.

Kamath MV, Fallen EL (1991) Diurnal variations of neurocardiac rhythms in acute myocardial infarction. Am J Cardiol 68:155-160.

Kamath MV, Fallen EL (1993) Power spectral analysis of heart rate variability: A noninvasive signature of cardiac autonomic function. Critical Rev in Biomed Eng 21:245-311.

Karason K, Molgaard H, Wikstrand J, Sjostrom L (1999) Heart rate variability in obesity and the effect of weight loss. Am J Cardiol 83:1242-1247.

Kaufman MP, Baker DG, Coleridge HM, Coleridge JCG (1980) Stimulation by bradykinin of afferent vagal C-fibers with chemosensitive endings in the heart and aorta of the dog. Circ Res 46:476-484.

Kawada T, Ikeda Y, Sugimachi M, Shishido T, Kawaguchi O, Yamazaki T, Alexander J Jr., Sunagawa K (1996) Bidirectional augmentation of heart rate regulation by autonomic nervous system in rabbits. Am J Physiol 271;H288-H295.

Kawada T, Sugimachi M, Shishido T, Miyano H, Ikeda Y, Yoshimura R, Sato T, Takaki H, Alexander J Jr., Sunagawa K (1997) Dynamic vagosympathetic interaction augments heart rate response irrespective of stimulation patterns. Am J Physiol 272;H2180-H2187.

Kerzner J, Wolf M, Kosowsky BD, Lown B (1973) Ventricular ectopic rhythms following vagal stimulation in dog with acute myocardial infarction. Circulation 47:44-50.

Kingwell BA, Thompson JM, Kaye DM, McPherson GA, Jennings GL, Esler MD (1994) Heart rate spectral analysis, cardiac norepinephrine spillover, and muscle sympathetic nerve activity during human sympathetic nervous activation and failure. Circulation 90:234-240.

Kitney RI, Byrne S, Edmonds ME, Watkins PJ, Roberts VC (1982) Heart rate variability in the assessment of autonomic diabetic neuropathy. Automedica 4:155-167.

Kitney RI, Bignall S (1993) Techniques for studying short-term changes in cardio-respiratory data. In: Di Rienzo M, et al. (eds) Blood pressure and heart rate variability, IOS Press, Amsterdam, pp 1-23.

Kitney R, Linkens D, Selman A, McDonald A (1982) The interaction between heart rate and respiration: Part II. Nonlinear analysis based on computer modelling. Automedica 4:141-153.

Kleiger RE, Miller JP, Bigger JT, Moss AR, Multicenter Post-infarction Research Group (1987) Decreased heart rate variability and its association with increased mortality after acute myocardial infarction. Am J Cardiol 59:256-262.

Kobayashi M, Musha T (1982) 1/f fluctuations of heartbeat period. IEEE Trans Biomed Eng 29:456-464.

Koepchen HP (1984) History of studies and concepts of blood pressure waves. In: Miyakawa K, Koepchen HP, Polosa CL (eds): Mechanisms of blood pressure waves. Tokyo/Berlin, Japanese Science Society Press/Springer Verlag, pp. 3-23.

Koepchen HP, Klüssendorf D, Sommer D (1981) Neurophysiological background of central neural cardiovascular-respiratory coordination: basic remarks and experimental approach. J Auton Nerv Syst 3:335-368.

Koh J, Brown TE, Beightol LA, Ha CY, Eckberg DL (1994) Human autonomic rhythms: vagal cardiac mechanisms in tetraplegic subjects. J Physiol (Lond) 474:483-495.

Kollai M, Koizumi K (1981) Cardiovascular reflexes and interrelationships between sympathetic and parasympathetic activity. J Autonom Nerv Syst 4:135-148.

Kontos H, Richardson DW, Norvell JE (1975) Norepinephrine depletion in idiopatic orthostatic hypotension. Ann Intern Med 82:336-341.

Kuhn TS (1970) The structure of scientific revolutions, Univ. Chicago Press.

Kumada N, Nogami K, Sagawa K (1975) Modulation of carotid sinus baroreceptor reflex by sciatic nerve stimulation. Am J Physiol 228:1535-1541.

Kunze DL (1975) Reflex discharge patterns of cardiac vagal efferent fibres. J Physiol (Lond) 222:1-15.

Lakatos I (1978) Philosophical papers, vol II, Cambridge Univ. Press.

Landsberg L (1986) Diet, obesity and hypertension: an hypothesis involving insulin, the sympathetic nervous system, and adaptive thermogenesis. Q J Med 61:1081-1090.

Langley JN (1896) Observation on the medullated fibres of the sympathetic system and chiefly on those of the grey rami communicantes. J Physiol (Lond) 20: 55-76.

Langley JN (1898) On the union of the cranial autonomic (visceral) fibres with the nerve cells of the superior cervical ganglion. J Physiol (Lond) 23: 240-270.

Langley JN (1903) The autonomic nervous system. Brain 26: 1-26.

Langley JN (1915-1916) Sketch of the progress of discovery in the eighteenth century as regards the autonomic nervous system. J Physiol (Lond) 50: 225-258.

Langley JN (1924) Vaso-motor centres. Part III Spinal vascular (and other autonomic) reflexes and the effect of strychnine on them. J Physiol (Lond) 59:231-258.

Lazzeri C, La Villa G, Mannelli M, Janni L, Barletta G, Montano N, Franchi F (1998) Effects of clonidine on power spectral analysis of heart rate variability in mild essential hypertension. J Autonom Nerv Syst 74:152-159.

La Rovere MT, Bigger JT, Marcus FI, Mortara A, Schwartz PJ (1998) Baroreflex sensitivity and heart-rate variability in prediction of total cardiac mortality after myocardial infarction. Lancet 351:478-484.

Legramante JM, Raimondi G, Massaro M, Cassarino S, Peruzzi G, Iellamo F (1999) Investigating feed-forward neural regulation of circulation from analysis of spontaneous arterial pressure and heart rate fluctuation. Circulation 99:1760-1766.

Lembo G, Capaldo B, Rendina V, Iaccarino G, Napoli T, Guida R, Trimarco B, Saccà L (1994) Acute noradrenergic activation induces insulin resistance in human skeletal muscles. Am J Physiol 266:E242-E247.

Le Pape G, Giacomini H, Swynghedauw B, Mansier P (1997) A statistical analysis of sequences of cardiac interbeat intervals does not support the chaos hypothesis. J Theor Biol 184:123-131.

Lepicovska V, Novak P, Nadeau R (1992) Time-frequency dynamics in neurally mediated syncope. Clin Autonom Res 2:317-326.

Levy MN (1971) Sympathetic-parasympathetic interactions in the heart. Circ Res 29:437-445.

Lewis T (1931) Angina pectoris associated with high blood pressure and its relief by amyl nitrite; with a note on Nothnagel's syndrome. Heart 15: 305-327.

Lewis T (1932a) Pain in muscular ischemia – its relation to anginal pain. Arch Intern Med 49: 713-727.

Lewis T (1932b) Vasovagal syncope and the carotid sinus mechanism with comments on Gowers's and Nothnagel's syndrome. Br Med J i:873-876.

Lewis T, Kellegren JH (1939-1942) Observation relating to referred pain, visceromotor reflexes and other associated phenomena. Clin Sci 4:47-71.

Lindgren I, Olivecrona H (1947) Surgical treatment of angina pectoris. J Neurosurg 4: 19-39.

Lioy F, Szeto PM (1975) Baroreceptor and chemoreceptor influence on the cardiovascular responses initiated by stretch of the thoracic aorta. Physiologist 18:293.

Lioy F, Malliani A, Pagani M, Recordati G, Schwartz PJ (1974) Reflex hemodynamic responses initiated from the thoracic aorta. Circ Res 34:78-84.

Lipsitz LA, Mietus J, Moody GB, Goldberger AL (1990) Spectral characteristics of heart rate variability before and during postural tilt. Circulation 81:1803-1810.

Lishner M, Akselrod S, Mor Avi V, Oz O, Divon M, Ravid M (1987) Spectral analysis of heart rate fluctuations. A non-invasive, sensitive method for the early diagnosis of autonomic neuropathy in diabetes mellitus. J Auton Nerv Syst 19:119-125.

Littler WA, Honour J, Sleight P, Stott FD (1973) Direct arterial pressure and electrocardiogram in unrestricted patients with angina pectoris. Circulation 48:125-134.

Lloyd-Mostyn RH, Watkins PJ (1976) Total cardiac denervation in diabetic autonomic neuropathy. Diabetes 25:748-751.

Lombardi F (1999) Heart rate variability: a contribution to a better understanding of the clinical role of heart rate. Europ Heart J 1 (suppl H): H44-H51.

Lombardi F, Malliani A, Pagani M (1976) Nervous activity of afferent sympathetic fibers innervating the pulmonary veins. Brain Res, 113:197-200.

Lombardi F, Della Bella P, Casati R, Malliani A (1981) Effects of intracoronary administration of bradykinin on the impulse activity of afferent sympathetic unmyelinated fibers with left ventricular endings in the cat. Circ Res 48:69-75.

Lombardi F, Patton CP, Della Bella P, Pagani M, Malliani A (1982) Cardiovascular and sympathetic responses reflexly elicited through the excitation with bradykinin of sympathetic and vagal cardiac sensory endings in the cat. Cardiovasc Res 16:57-65

Lombardi F, Casalone C, Della Bella P, Malfatto, Pagani M, Malliani A (1984) Global versus regional myocardial ischaemia: differences in cardiovascular and sympathetic responses in cats. Cardiovasc Res 18:14-23.

Lombardi F, Casalone C, Malfatto G, Gnecchi Ruscone T, Casati R, Malliani A (1986) Effects of propranolol on the impulse activity of cardiovascular sympathetic afferent fibers. Hypertension 8:50-55.

Lombardi F, Sandrone G, Pernpruner S, Sala R, Garimoldi M, Cerutti S, Baselli G, Pagani M, Malliani A (1987) Heart rate variability as an index of sympathovagal interaction after acute myocardial infarction. Am J Cardiol 60:1239-1245.

Lombardi F, Gnecchi Ruscone T, Malliani A (1989) Premature ventricular contractions and reflex sympathetic activation in cats. Cardiovasc Res 23:205-212.

Lombardi F, Sandrone G, Mortara A, La Rovere MT, Colombo E, Guzzetti S, Malliani A (1992) Circadian variation of spectral indices of heart rate variability after myocardial infarction. Am Heart J 123:1521-1529.

Lombardi F, Malliani A, Pagani M, Cerutti S (1996a) Heart rate variability and its sympatho-vagal modulation. Cardiovasc Res 32:208-216.

Lombardi F, Sandrone G, Mortara A, Torzillo D, La Rovere MT, Signorini MG, Cerutti S, Malliani A (1996b) Linear and nonlinear dyamics of heart rate variability after acute myocardial infarction with normal and reduced left ventricular ejection fraction. Am J Cardiol 77:1283-1288.

Lombardi F, Sandrone G, Spinnler MT, Torzillo D, Lavezzaro GC, Brusca A, Malliani A (1996c) Heart rate variability in the early hours of an acute myocardial infarction. Am J Cardiol 77:1037-1044.

Low PA, Opfer-Gehrking TL, Textor SC, Bernarroch EE, Shen WK, Schondorf R, Suarez GA, Rummans TA (1995) Postural tachycardia syndrome (POTS). Neurology 45:S19-S25.

Lown B (1979) Sudden cardiac death: The major challenge confronting contemporary cardiology. Am J Cardiol 43:313-328.

Lown B (1996) The lost art of healing. Houghton Mifflin, Boston.

Lown B, Verrier RL (1976) Neural activity and ventricular fibrillation. N Engl J Med 294:1165-1170.

Lown B, Fakhro AM, Hood WB Jr, Thorn GW (1967) The coronary care unit: new perspectives and directions. J Am Med Ass 199:188-198.

Lucini D, Pagani M, Mela GS, Malliani A (1994) Sympathetic restraint of baroreflex control of heart period in normotensive and hypertensive subjects. Clin Sci 86:547-556.

Ma R, Zucker IH, Wang W (1997) Central gain of the cardiac sympathetic afferent reflex in dogs with heart failure. Am J Physiol 273:H2664-H2671.

Maayan C, Axelrod FB, Akselrod S, Carley DW, Shannon CD (1987) Evaluation of autonomic dysfunction in familial dysautonomia by power spectral analysis. J Autonom Nerv Syst 21:51-58.

Makino Y, Kawano Y, Okuda N, Horio T, Iwashima N, Yamada N, Takamiya M, Takishita S (1999) Autonomic function in hypertensive patients with neurovascular compression of the ventrolateral medulla oblongata. J Hypertens 17:1257-1263.

Malik M, Camm AJ (1993) Components of heart rate variability. What they really mean and what we really measure. Am J Cardiol 72:821-822.

Malik M, Camm AJ (eds.) (1995) Heart rate variability. Armonk, NY. Futura Publishing Company, Inc.

Malliani A (1979) Afferent cardiovascular sympathetic fibres and their function in the neural regulation of the circulation. In: Cardiac receptors, Hainsworth R, Kidd C and Linden JR (eds), Cambridge University Press, Cambridge, pp 319-338.

Malliani A (1980) Disagreement on the reflex sympathetic activity elicited by experimental coronary occlusion. Circ Res 47:627-628.

Malliani A (1982) Cardiovascular sympathetic afferent fibers. Rev Physiol Biochem Pharmacol 94: 11-74.

Malliani A (1986) The elusive link between transient myocardial ischemia and pain. Circulation 73:201-204.

Malliani A (1995) Association of heart rate variability components with physiological regulatory mechanisms. In: Heart rate variability. Malik M, Camm AJ (eds.) Armonk, NY, Futura Publishing Company Inc., pp. 173-188.

Malliani A (1997) The autonomic nervous system: A Sherringtonian revision of its integrated properties in the control of circulation. J Auton Nerv Syst 64:158-161.

Malliani A (1999a) The pattern of sympathovagal balance explored in the frequency domain. News Physiol Sci 14:111-117.

Malliani A (1999b) Ethical aspects of clinical practice. Europ J Intern Med 10:76-81.

Malliani A, Brown AM (1970) Reflex arising from coronary receptors. Brain Res 24:352-355.

Malliani A, Lombardi F (1982) Consideration of the fundamental mechanisms eliciting cardiac pain. Am Heart J 103: 575-578.

Malliani A, Pagani M (1976) Afferent sympathetic nerve fibres with aortic endings. J Physiol (Lond) 263:157-169.

Malliani A, Pagani M (1983) The role of the sympathetic nervous system in congestive heart failure. Europ Heart J 4(suppl A):49-54.

Malliani A, Schwartz PJ, Zanchetti A (1969) A sympathetic reflex elicited by experimental coronary occlusion. Am J Physiol 217:703-709

Malliani A, Pagani M, Recordati G, Schwartz PJ (1971) Spinal sympathetic reflexes elicited by increases in arterial blood pressure. Am J Physiol 220:128-134.

Malliani A, Peterson DF, Bishop VS, Brown AM (1972) Spinal sympathetic cardiovascular reflexes. Circ Res 30:158-166.

Malliani A, Parks M, Tuckett RP, Brown AM (1973a) Reflex increases in heart rate elicited by stimulation of afferent cardiac sympathetic nerve fibers in the cat. Circ Res 32: 9-14.

Malliani A, Recordati G, Schwartz PJ (1973b) Nervous activity of afferent cardiac sympathetic fibres with atrial and ventricular endings. J Physiol (Lond) 229:457-469.

Malliani A, Lombardi F, Pagani M, Recordati G, Schwartz PJ (1975a) Spinal cardiovascular reflexes. Brain Res 87: 239-246.

Malliani A, Lombardi F, Pagani M, Recordati G, Schwartz PJ (1975b) Spinal sympathetic reflexes in the cat and the pathogenesis of arterial hypertension. Clin Sci Molec Med 48:259s-260s.

Malliani A, Pagani M, Bergamaschi M (1979) Positive feedback sympathetic reflexes and hypertension. Am J Cardiol 44: 860-865.

Malliani A, Schwartz PJ, Zanchetti A (1980) Neural mechanisms in life-threatening arrhythmias. Am Heart J 100:705-715.

Malliani A, Lombardi F, Pagani M (1986a) Sensory innervation of the heart. In Cervero F, Morrison JFB (eds.): Progress in Brain Reserarch, Vol. 67, Amsterdam, Elsevier Science Publishers B.V., pp. 39-48.

Malliani A, Pagani M, Lombardi F (1986b) Positive feedback reflexes. In Zanchetti A, Tarazi RC (eds): Handbook of hypertension, Vol. 8, Amsterdam, Elsevier Science Publishers B.V., pp 69-81.

Malliani A, Pagani M, Lombardi F (1989) Visceral versus somatic mechanisms. In Wall PD Melzack R (eds.), Textbook of Pain, 2nd edition, Churchill Livingstone Edinburgh pp.128-140.

Malliani A, Pagani M, Lombardi F, Cerutti S (1991a) Cardiovascular neural regulation explored in the frequency domain. Research Advances Series, Circulation 84:482-492.

Malliani A, Pagani M, Lombardi F, Furlan R, Guzzetti S, Cerutti S (1991b) Spectral analysis to assess increased sympathetic tone in arterial hypertension. Hypertension 17:III36-III42.

Malliani A, Lombardi F, Pagani M, Cerutti S (1994a) Power spectral analysis of cardiovascular variability in patients at risk for sudden cardiac death. J Cardiovasc Electrophysiol 5:274-286.

Malliani A, Pagani M, Lombardi F (1994b) Methods for assessment of sympatho-vagal balance: power spectral analysis. In: Vagal control of the heart: experimental basis and clinical implications. Levy MN, Schwartz PJ (eds), Futura Publishing Co. Inc., Armonk, NY, pp 433-454.

Malliani A, Montano N, Pagani M (1997a) Physiological background of heart rate variability. Cardiac Electrophysiol Rev 1:343-346.

Malliani A, Pagani M, Furlan R, Guzzetti S, Lucini D, Montano N, Cerutti S, Mela GS (1997b) Individual recognition by heart rate variability of two different autonomic profiles related to posture. Circulation 96:4143-4145.

Malliani A, Pagani M, Montano N, Mela GS (1998) Sympathovagal balance: A reappraisal. Circulation 98:2640-2644.

Mancia G (1990) Sympathetic activation in congestive heart failure. Eur Heart J 11(suppl.A): 3-11.

Mannheimer C, Carlsson CA, Vedin A, Wilhelmsson C (1986) Transcutaneous electrical nerve stimulation (TENS) in angina pectoris. Pain 26: 291-300.

Mansier P, Clairambault J, Charlotte N, Médigue C, Vermeiren C, LePape G, Carré F, Gounaropoulou A, Swynghedauw B (1996a) Linear and non-linear analyses of heart rate variability: a minireview. Cardiovasc Res 31:371-379.

Mansier P, Médigue C, Charlotte N, Vermeiren C, Coraboeuf E, Deroubai E, Ratner E, Chevalier B, Clairambault J, Carré F, Dahkli T, Bertin B, Briand P, Strosberg D, Swynghedauw B (1996b) Decreased heart rate variability in transgenic mice overexpressing atrial β1-adrenoceptors. Am J Physiol 271:H1465-H1472.

Martin SJ, Gorham LW (1938) Cardiac Pain. An experimental study with reference to the tension factor. Arch Intern Med 62:840-852.

Maseri A, Severi S, De Nes M, L'Abbate A, Chierchia S, Marzilli M, Ballestra AM, Parodi O, Biagini A, Distante A (1978) Variant angina: one aspect of a continuous spectrum of vasospastic myocardial ischemia. Am J Cardiol 42:1019-1035.

Maseri A, Chierchia S, Davies G, Glazier J (1985) Mechanisms of ischemic cardiac pain and silent myocardial ischemia. Am J Med 79:7-11.

Mathias CJ, Frankel HL (1988) Cardiovascular control in spinal man. Ann Rev Physiol 50:577-592.

Mayer S (1876) Studien zur Physiologie des Herzens und der Blutgefässe: 5. Abhandlung: Über spontane Blutdruck-schwankungen. Sber. Akad Wiss. Wien, 3 Abt. 74:281-307.

Mc Dermott W (1971) Medicine in modern society. In: Cecil-Loeb Textbook of Medicine, 13th edition, W.B. Saunders Co., Philadelphia, pp. 1-3.

Minisi AJ, Thames AD (1991) Activation of cardiac sympathetic afferents during coronary occlusion: Evidence for reflex activation of the sympathetic nervous system during transmural myocardial ischemia in the dog. Circulation 84:357-367.

Miyakawa K, Koepchen HP, Polosa CL (1984) Mechanisms of blood pressure waves. Tokyo/Berlin, Japanese Science Society Press/Springer Verlag, pp. 43-56.

Montano N, Lombardi F, Gnecchi Ruscone T, Contini M, Finocchiaro ML, Baselli G, Porta A, Cerutti S, Malliani A (1992) Spectral analysis of sympathetic discharge, R-R interval and systolic arterial pressure in decerebrate cats. J Autonom Nerv Syst 40:21-32

Montano N, Gnecchi Ruscone T, Porta A, Lombardi F, Pagani M, Malliani A (1994) Power spectrum analysis of heart rate variability to assess the changes in sympathovagal balance during graded orthostatic tilt. Circulation 90:1826-1831.

Montano N, Gnecchi Ruscone T, Porta A, Lombardi F, Malliani A (1996a) Occurrence in the discharge of the isolated sympathetic spinal outflow of a rhythmicity in phase with vasomotor activity. XVIII Congress of the European Society of Cardiology. Birmingham, U.K., August 25-29, P1035.

Montano N, Gnecchi Ruscone T, Porta A, Lombardi F, Malliani A, Barman SM (1996b) Presence of vasomotor and respiratory rhythms in the discharge of single medullary neurons involved in the regulation of cardiovascular system. J Autonom Nerv Syst 57:116-122.

Montano N, Cogliati C, Porta A, Pagani M, Malliani A, Narkyewicz C, Abboud FM, Birkett C, Somers VK (1998) Central vagotonic effects of atropine modulate spectral oscillations of sympathetic nerve activity. Circulation 98:1394-1399.

Morillo CA, Klein GJ, Jones DL, Yee R (1994) Time and frequency domain analyses of heart rate variability during orthostatic stress in patients with neurally mediated syncope. Am J Cardiol 74:1258-1262.

Mortara A, Sleight P, Pinna GD, Maestri R, Prpa A, La Rovere MT, Cobelli F, Tavazzi L (1997) Abnormal awake respiratory patterns are common in chronic heart failure and may prevent evaluation of autonomic tone by measures of heart rate variability. Circulation 96:246-252.

Moruzzi G (1940) Paleocerebellar inhibition of vasomotor and respiratory carotid sinus reflexes. J Neurophysiol 3:20-32.

Müller J (1840) Handbuch der Physiologie des Menschen für Vorlesungen. Hollscher, Koblenz.

Muller JE, Tofler GH, Stone PH (1989) Circadian variation and triggers of onset of acute cardiovascular disease. Circulation 79:733-743.

Murphy DF, Giles KE (1987) Dorsal column stimulation for pain relief from intractable angina pectoris. Pain 28:365-368.

Narkiewicz K, Somers VK (1998) Chronic orthostatic intolerance. Part of a spectrum of dysfunction in orthostatic cardiovascular homeostasis? Circulation 98:2105-2107.

Narkiewicz K, Montano N, Cogliati C, van de Borne PJ, Dyken ME, Somers VK (1998) Altered cardiovascular variability in obstructive sleep apnea. Circulation 98:1071-1077.

Neto FR, Brasil JCF, Antonio A (1974) Bradykinin induced coronary chemoreflex in the dog. Arch Exp Pathol Pharmakol 283:135-142.

Neufeld HN, Zivner Z, Eldar M, Rabinowitz B. (1978) Sinus bradycardia in acute myocardial infarction. In: Schwartz PJ, Brown AM, Malliani A, Zanchetti A (eds.) Neural mechanisms in cardiac arrhythmias, Raven Press, New York, pp 19-30.

Nishi K, Sakanashi M, Takenaka F (1977) Activation of afferent cardiac sympathetic nerve fibres of the cat by pain producing substances and by noxious heat. Pfluegers Arch 372:53-61.

Nolan J, Batin PD, Andrews R, Lindsay SJ, Brooksby P, Mullen M, Baig W, Flapan AD, Cowley A, Prescott RJ, Neilson JMM, Fox KAA (1998) Prospective study of heart rate variability and mortality in chronic heart failure. Results of the United Kingdom heart failure evaluation and assessment of risk trial (UK-Heart). Circulation 98:1510-1516.

Nonidez JF (1941) Studies on the innervation of the heart. II. Afferent nerve endings in the large arteries and veins. Am J Anat 68:151-189.

Öberg B, Thorén P (1972) Increased activity in left ventricular receptors during hemorrhage or occlusion of caval veins in the cat. A possible cause of the vaso-vagal reaction. Acta Physiol Scand 85:164-173.

Osler W (1910) The Lumleian lectures on 'angina pectoris' (lecture II). Lancet i: 839-844.

Packer M (1998) β-adrenergic blockade in chronic heart failure: principles, progress, and practice. Progr Cardiovasc Dis 41:39-52.

Pagani M, Schwartz PJ, Banks R, Lombardi F, Malliani A (1974) Reflex responses of sympathetic preganglionic neurones initiated by different cardiovascular receptors in spinal animals. Brain Res. 68:215-225.

Pagani M, Schwartz PJ, Bishop VS, Malliani A (1975) Reflex sympathetic changes in the aortic diastolic pressure-diameter relationship. Am J Physiol 229:286-290.

Pagani M, Mirsky I, Baig H, Manders WT, Kerkof P, Vatner SF (1979) Effects of age on aortic pressure-diameter and elastic stiffness-stress relationship in unanesthetized sheep. Circ Res 44:420-429.

Pagani M, Pizzinelli P, Bergamaschi M, Malliani A (1982) A positive feedback sympathetic pressor reflex during stretch of the thoracic aorta in conscious dogs. Circ Res 50:125-132.

Pagani M, Furlan R, Dell'Orto S, Pizzinelli P, Baselli G, Cerutti S, Lombardi F, Malliani A (1985a) Simultaneous analysis of beat by beat systemic arterial pressure and heart rate variabilities in ambulatory patients. J Hypertens 3:S83-S85.

Pagani M, Pizzinelli P, Furlan F, Guzzetti S, Rimoldi O, Sandrone G, Malliani A (1985b) Analysis of the pressor sympathetic reflex produced by intracoronary injections of bradykinin in conscious dogs. Circ Res 56:175-183.

Pagani M, Furlan R, Dell'Orto S, Pizzinelli P, Lanzi G, Baselli G, Santoli C, Cerutti S, Lombardi F, Malliani A (1986a) Continuous recording of direct high fidelity arterial pressure and electrocardiogram in unrestricted subjects. Cardiovasc Res 20:384-388.

Pagani M, Lombardi F, Guzzetti S, Rimoldi O, Furlan R, Pizzinelli P, Sandrone G, Malfatto G, Dell'Orto S, Piccaluga E, Turiel M, Baselli G, Cerutti S, Malliani A (1986b) Power spectral analysis of heart rate and arterial pressure variabilities as a marker of sympathovagal interaction in man and conscious dog. Circ Res 58:178-193.

Pagani M, Malfatto G, Pierini S, Casati R, Masu AM, Poli M, Guzzetti S, Lombardi F, Cerutti S, Malliani A (1988a) Spectral analysis of heart rate variability in the assessment of autonomic diabetic neuropathy. J Autonom Nerv Syst 23:143-153

Pagani M, Somers VK, Furlan R, Dell'Orto S, Conway J, Baselli G, Cerutti S, Sleight P, Malliani A (1988b) Changes in autonomic regulation induced by physical training in mild hypertension. Hypertension 12:600-610.

Pagani M, Furlan R, Pizzinelli P, Crivellaro W, Cerutti S, Malliani A (1989) Spectral analysis of R-R and arterial pressure variabilities to assess sympatho-vagal interaction during mental stress in humans. J Hypertens 7 (suppl 6):S14-S15.

Pagani M, Mazzuero G, Ferrari A, Liberati D, Cerutti S, Vaitl D, Tavazzi L, Malliani A (1991) Sympathovagal interaction during mental stress. A study employing spectral analysis of heart rate variability in healthy control subjects and patients with prior myocardial infarction. Circulation 83(suppl II):II-43-II-51

Pagani M, Lombardi F, Malliani A (1993) Heart rate variability: disagreement on the markers of sympathetic and parasympathetic activities. J Am Coll Cardiol 22:951-954.

Pagani M, Lucini D, Mela GS, Langewitz W, Malliani A (1994) Sympathetic overactivity in subjects complaining of unexplained fatigue. Clin Sci 87:655-661.

Pagani M, Lucini D, Pizzinelli P, Sergi M, Bosisio E, Mela GS, Malliani A (1996) Effects of aging and of chronic obstructive pulmonary disease on RR interval variability. J Autonom Nerv Syst 59:125-132.

Pagani M, Montano N, Porta A, Malliani A, Abboud FM, Birkett C, Somers VK (1997) Relationship between spectral components of cardiovascular variabilities and direct measures of muscle sympathetic nerve activity in humans. Circulation 95:1441-1448.

Page IH (1949) Pathogenesis of arterial hypertension. J Am Med Ass 140:451-457.

Page IH, McCubbin JW, Corcoran AC (1958) Guide to the theory of arterial hypertension. Perspect Biol Med 1:307-325.

Paintal AS (1971) Action of drugs on sensory nerve endings. Ann Rev Pharmacol 11: 231-240.

Palatini P, Mos L, Mormino P, Di Marco A, Munari L, Fazio G, Giuliano G, Pessina AC, Dal Palù C (1989) Blood pressure changes during running in humans: the "beat" phenomenon. J Appl Physiol 67:52-59.

Palmer RM, Ferrige AG, Moncada S (1987) Nitric oxide release accounts for the biologic activity of endothelium-derived relaxing factor. Nature 327:524-526.

Pantridge JF (1978) Autonomic disturbance at the onset of acute myocardial infarction. In: Schwartz PJ, Brown AM, Malliani A, Zanchetti A (eds) Neural mechanisms in cardiac arrhythmias. Raven Press, New York, pp 7-17.

Pantridge JF, Webb SW, Adgey AAJ (1981) Arrhythmias in the first hours of acute myocardial infarction. Prog Cardiovasc Dis 23:265-278.

Parati G, Castiglioni P, Di Rienzo M, Omboni S, Pedotti A, Mancia G (1990) Sequential spectral analysis of 24-hour blood pressure and pulse interval in humans. Hypertension 16:414-421.

Parati G, Di Rienzo M, Groppelli A, Pedotti A, Mancia G (1995a) Heart rate and blood pressure variability and their interaction in hypertension. In: Heart rate variability. Malik M, Camm AJ (eds.) Armonk, NY, Futura Publishing Company Inc., pp 467-478.

Parati G, Saul JP, Di Rienzo M, Mancia G (1995b) Spectral analysis of blood pressure and heart rate variability in evaluating cardiovascular regulation. A critical appraisal. Hypertension 25:1276-1286.

Pellegrino ED, Relman AS (1999) Professional Medical Associations: Ethical and practical guidelines. J Am Med Ass 282:984-986.

Perl ER (1971) Is pain a specific sensation? J Psychiatr Res 8:273-287.

Persson PB, Wagner CD (1996) General principles of chaotic dynamics. Cardiovasc Res 31:332-341.

Peterson DF, Brown AM (1971) Pressor reflexes produced by stimulation of afferent cardiac nerve fibres in the cardiac sympathetic nerves of the cat. Circ Res 28: 605-610.

Piazza S, Furlan R, Dell'Orto S, Porta A, Lombardi F, Pagani M, Malliani A (1995) Mechanical effects of respiration and stepping on systolic arterial pressure variability during treadmill exercise. J Hypertens 13:1643-1647.

Piccirillo G, Bucca C, Durante M, Santagada E, Munizzi MR, Cacciafesta M, Marigliano V (1996) Heart rate and blood pressure variabilities in salt-sensitive hypertension. Hypertension 28:944-952.

Pickering G (1961) The nature of essential hypertension. Churchill Livingstone, London.

Pickering G (1978) Normotension and hypertension: the mysterious viability of the false. Am J Med 65:561-563.

Pikkujämsä SM, Mäkikallio TH, Sourander LB, Räihä IJ, Puukka P, Skyttä J, Peng CK, Goldberger AL, Huikuri HV (1999) Cardiac interbeat interval dynamics from childhood to senescence. Comparison of conventional and new measures based on fractals and chaos theory. Circulation 100:393-399.

Pincus SM (1991) Approximated entropy as a measure of system complexity. Proc Natl Acad Sci USA 88:2297-2311.

Pitzalis MV, Mastropasqua F, Massari F, Forleo C, Di Maggio M, Passantino A, Colombo R, Di Biase M, Rizzon P (1996) Short- and long-term reproducibility of time and frequency domain heart rate variability measurements in normal subjects. Cardiovasc Res 32:226-233.

Polosa C (1984) Central nervous system origin of some types of Mayer waves. In: Miyakawa K, Koepchen HP, Polosa CL (eds): Mechanisms of blood pressure waves. Tokyo/Berlin, Japanese Science Society Press/Springer Verlag, pp. 277-292.

Pomeranz B, Macaulay RJB, Caudill MA, Kutz I, Adam D, Gordon D, Kilborn KM, Barger AC, Shannon DC, Cohen RJ, Benson H (1985) Assessment of autonomic function in humans by heart rate spectral analysis. Am J Physiol 248:H151-H153.

Ponikowski P, Anker SD, Chua TP, Szelemej R, Piepoli M, Adamopoulos S, Webb-Peploe K, Harrington D, Banasiak W, Wrabec K, Coats AJ (1997) Depressed heart rate variability as an independent predictor of death in chronic congestive heart failure secondary to ischemic or idiopathic dilated cardiomyopathy. Am J Cardiol 79:1645-1650.

Porta A (1998) Multivariate method based on conditional entropy estimate for measuring regularity, synchronisation and coordination in cardiovascular variability signals. PhD Thesis, Dipartimento di Bioingegneria, Politecnico di Milano.

Porta A, Baselli G, Manessi E, Manziana A, Cerutti S, Montano N, Gnecchi Ruscone T, Lombardi F, Malliani A (1995) Different interference patterns among spontaneous low and high frequency oscillations and forced ventilation in sympathetic outflow. Comput Cardiol 473-476.

Porta A, Baselli G, Montano N, Gnecchi Ruscone T, Lombardi F, Malliani A, Cerutti S (1996) Classification of coupling patterns among spontaneous rhythms and ventilation in the sympathetic discharge of decerebrate cats. Biol Cybern 75:163-172.

Porta A, Baselli G, Guzzetti S, Magatelli R, Montano N, Cogliati C, Malliani A, Cerutti S (1997) Synchronisation analysis of heart rate period variability signal based on corrected conditional entropy. Comp Cardiol 24:121-124.

Porta A, Baselli G, Liberati D, Montano N, Cogliati C, Gnecchi Ruscone T, Malliani A, Cerutti S (1998) Measuring regularity by means of a corrected conditional entropy in sympathetic outflow. Biol Cybern 78:71-78.

Porta A, Baselli G, Lombardi F, Montano N, Malliani A, Cerutti S (1999) Conditional entropy approach for the evaluation of the coupling strength. Biol Cybern 81:119-129.

Porta A, Guzzetti S, Montano N, Pagani M, Somers V, Malliani A, Baselli G, Cerutti S (2000) Information domain analysis of cardiovascular variability signals: evaluation of regularity, synchronisation and coordination. Med Biol Eng Comp (in press).

Preiss G, Polosa C (1974) Patterns of sympathetic neuron activity associated with Mayer waves. Am J Physiol 226:724-730.

Procacci P, Zoppi M (1989) Heart pain. In: Wall PD, Melzack R (eds) Texbook of pain, 2nd edn. Churchill Livingstone, Edinburgh, pp 410-419.

Procacci P, Zoppi M, Padeletti L, Maresca M (1976) Myocardial infarction without pain. A study of the sensory functions of the upper limbs. Pain 2: 309-313.

Radaelli A, Bernardi L, Valle F, Leuzzi S, Salvucci F, Pedrotti L, Marchesi E, Finardi G, Sleight P (1994) Cardiovascular autonomic modulation in essential hypertension. Effect of tilting. Hypertension 24:556-563.

Randall WC, McNally H, Cowan J, Caliguiri L, Rohse WG (1957) Functional analysis of the cardioaugmentor and cardioaccelerator pathways in the dog. Am J Physiol 191:213-217.

Recordati G (1984) The functional role of the visceral nervous system. A critical evaluation of Cannon's "homeostatic" and "emergency" theories. Arch Ital Biol 122: 249-267.

Recordati G, Schwartz PJ, Pagani M, Malliani A, Brown AM (1971) Activation of cardiac vagal receptors during myocardial ischaemia. Experientia 27:1423-1424.

Reid MR, De Witt A (1925) The surgical treatment of angina pectoris. Ann Surg 81:591-604.

Reinmann KA, Weaver LC (1980) Contrasting reflexes evoked by chemical activation of cardiac afferent nerves. Am J Physiol 239:H316-H325.

Rimoldi O, Pierini S, Ferrari A, Cerutti S, Pagani M, Malliani A (1990) Analysis of short-term oscillations of RR and arterial pressure in conscious dogs. Am J Physiol 258:H967-H976.

Rimoldi O, Furlan R, Pagani MR, Piazza S, Guazzi M, Pagani M, Malliani A (1992) Analysis of neural mechanisms accompanying different intensities of dynamic exercise. Chest 101:226S-230S.

Rimoldi O, Pagani MR, Piazza S, Pagani M, Malliani A (1994) Restraining effects of captopril on sympathetic excitatory responses in dogs. Am J Physiol 267:H1608-H1618.

Rinzler SH (1952) Cardiac pain. Charles C Thomas, Springfield, Ill.

Roach D, Malik M, Koshman ML, Sheldon R (1999) Origins of heart rate variability. Inducibility and prevalence of a discrete, tachycardic event. Circulation 99:3279-3285.

Robbe HWJ, Mulder JM, Rüddel H, Langewitz WA, Veldman JBP, Mulder G (1987) Assessment of baroreceptor reflex sensitivity by means of spectral analysis. Hypertension 10:538-543.

Robertson D, Hollister AS, Forman MB, Robertson RM (1985) Reflexes unique to myocardial ischemia and infarction. J Am Coll Cardiol 5:99B-104B.

Rose SPR (1998) Lifelines: Biology beyond determinism. Oxford Univ. Press., NY.

Roughgarden JW (1966) Circulatory changes associated with spontaneous angina pectoris. Am J Med 41:947-961.

Rubini R, Porta A, Baselli G, Cerutti S, Paro M (1993) Power spectrum analysis of cardiovascular variability monitored by telemetry in conscious unrestrained rats. J Autonom Nerv Syst 45:181-190.

Ruch TC (1955) Pathophysiology of pain. In Fulton JF (ed.), A texbook of physiology, WB Saunders Co, Philadelphia.

Rundqvist B, Elam M, Bergmann-Sverrisdottir Y, Eisenhofer G, Friberg P. (1997) Increased cardiac adrenergic drive precedes generalized sympathetic activation in human heart failure. Circulation 95:169-175.

Rushmer RF, Smith OA, Lasher EP (1960) Neural mechanisms of cardiac control during exertion. Physiol Rev (Suppl) 40: 27-34.

Sagawa K (1983) Baroreflex control of systemic arterial pressure and vascular bed. In: Shepherd JT, Abboud FM, Geiger SR (eds): Handbook of physiology, Section 2, The cardiovascular system, vol III. Peripheral circulation and organ blood flow. American Physiological Society, Washington, pp. 453-496.

Sandrone G, Mortara A, Torzillo D, La Rovere MT, Malliani A, Lombardi F (1994) Effects of beta blockers (atenolol or metoprolol) on heart rate variability after acute myocardial infarction. Am J Cardiol 74:340-345.

Sands KEF, Appel ML, Lilly LS, Schoen FJ, Mudge GH, Cohen RJ (1989) Power spectrum analysis of heart rate variability in human cardiac transplant recipients. 79:76-82.

Saul JP, Arai Y, Berger RD, Lilly LS, Colucci WS, Cohen RJ (1988) Assessment of autonomic regulation in chronic congestive heart failure by heart rate spectral analysis. Am J Cardiol 61:1292-1299.

Sayers B McA (1973) Analysis of heart rate variability. Ergonomics 16:17-32.

Schmidt G, Malik M, Barthel P, Schneider R, Ulm K, Rolnitzky L, Camm AJ, Bigger JT (1999) Heart-rate turbulence after ventricular premature beats as a predictor of mortality after acute myocardial infarction. Lancet 353:1390-1396.

Schrier RW, Abraham WT (1999) Hormones and hemodynamics in heart failure. N Engl J Med 341:577585.

Schwartz PJ, Pagani M, Lombardi F Malliani A, Brown AM (1973) A cardiocardiac sympathovagal reflex in the cat. Circ Res 32:215-220.

Selman A, McDonald A, Kitney R, Linkens D (1982) The interaction between heart rate and respiration: part I - experimental studies in man. Automedica 4:131-139

Sherrington CS (1898) Decerebrate rigidity, and reflex coordination of movements. J Physiol (Lond) 22: 319-332.

Sherrington CS (1906) The integrative action of the nervous system, Yale University Press, New Haven.

Sherrington CS (1929) Ferrier Lecture: Some functional problems attaching to convergence. Proc Roy Soc Ser B 105:332-362.

Shusterman V, Aysin B, Gottipaty V, Weiss R, Brode S, Schwartzman D, Anderson KP (1998) Autonomic nervous system activity and the spontaneous initiation of ventricular tachycardia. J Am Coll Cardiol 32:1891-1899.

Sica AL, Hundley BW, Ruggiero DA, Gootman PM (1997) Emergence of lung-inflation-related sympathetic nerve activity in spinal cord transected neonatal swine. Brain Res 767:380-383.

Singh JP, Larson MG, O'Donnel CJ, Tsuji H, Evans JC, Levy D (1999) Heritability of heart rate variability. The Framingham heart study. Circulation 99:2251-2254.

Singh N, Mironov D, Armstrong PW, Ross AM, Langer A (1996) Heart rate variability assessment early after acute myocardial infarction. Pathophysiological and prognostic correlates. Circulation 93:1388-1395.

Skrabanek P (1986) Demarcation of the absurd. Lancet 1:960-961.

Sleight P (1986) Disorders of neural control of the cardiovascular system: clinical implications of cardiovascular reflexes. In: Zanchetti A, Tarazi RC (eds): Handbook of hypertension, Vol. 8, Amsterdam, Elsevier Science Publisher B.V., pp. 82-95.

Sleight P, La Rovere MT, Mortara A, Pinna G, Maestri R, Leuzzi S, Bianchini B, Tavazzi L, Bernardi L (1995) Physiology and pathophysiology of heart rate and blood pressure variability in humans. Is power spectral analysis largely an index of baroreflex gain? Clin Sci 88:103-109.

Smith LH (1988) Medicine as an art. In: Cecil Textbook of Medicine, 18th edition, W.B. Saunders Co., Philadelphia, pp. 1-5.

Smith OA (1974) Reflex and central mechanisms involved in the control of the heart and circulation. Ann Rev Physiol 36: 9-123.

Smyth HS, Sleight P, Pickering GW (1969) Reflex regulation of arterial pressure during sleep in man. A quantitative method of assessing baroreflex sensitivity. Circ Res 24:109-121

Spyer KM (1990) The central nervous organization of reflex circulatory control. In: Central regulation of autonomic functions, Loewy AD and Spyer KM (eds), Oxford University Press, New York/Oxford, pp 168-188.

Staszewska-Barczak J, Ferreira SH, Vane JR (1976) An excitatory nociceptive catrdiac reflex elicited by bradykinin and potentiated by prostaglandins and myocardial ischaemia. Cardiovasc Res 10:314-327.

Streeten DHP (1990) Pathogenesis of hyperadrenergic orthostatic hypotension. J Clin Invest 86:1582-1588.

Sugihara G, Allan W, Sobel D, Allan KD (1996) Nonlinear control of heart rate variability in human infants. Proc Natl Acad Sci 93:2608-2613.

Sutton DC, Lueth HC (1930) Experimental production of pain on excitation of the heart and great vessels. Arch Intern Med 45: 827-867.

Sylvén C, Beermann B, Jonzon B, Brandt R (1986) Angina pectoris-like pain provoked by intravenous adenosine. Br Med J 293:227-230.

Takens F (1981) Detecting strange attractors in turbulence. In: Lecture Notes in Mathematics. New York/Heidelberg, Springer-Verlag, vol 898, pp 366-381.

Taquini AC, Aviado DM (1961) Reflex stimulation of heart induced by partial occlusion of pulmonary artery. Am J Physiol 200: 647-650.

Task Force of the European Society of Cardiology and the North American Society of Pacing and Electrophysiology (1996) Heart rate variability. Standards and measurement, physiological interpretation, and clinical use. Circulation 93:1043-1065.

Tennant R, Wiggers CJ (1935) The effect of coronary occlusion on myocardial contraction. Am J Physiol 112: 351-361.

Thames MD (1980) Effect of d- and l-propranolol on the discharge of cardiac vagal C fibers. Am J Physiol 238:H465-H470.

Thames MD, Klopfenstein HS, Abboud FM, Mark AL, Walker JL. (1978) Preferential distribution of inhibitory cardiac receptors with vagal afferents to the inferoposterior wall of the dog. Circ Res 43:512-519.

Theiler J, Eubank S, Longtin A, Galdrikian B (1992) Testing for nonlinearity in time series: the method of surrogate data. Physica D 58:77-94.

Thomas JA, Marks BH (1978) Plasma norepinephrine in congestive heart failure. Am J Cardiol 4:233-243.

Thorén P (1977) Characteristics of left ventricular receptors with non-medullated vagal afferents in cats. Circ Res 40:415-421.

Timio M, Verdecchia P, Venanzi S, Gentili S, Ronconi M, Francucci B, Montanari M, Bichisao E (1988) Age and blood pressure changes. A 20-year follow-up study in nuns in a secluded order. Hypertension 12:457-461.

Tougas G, Kamath M, Watteel G, Fitzpatrick D, Fallen EL, Hunt RH, Upton ARM (1997) Modulation of neurocardiac function by oesophageal stimulation in humans. Clinical Science 92:167-174.

Uchida Y, Murao S (1974a) Excitation of afferent cardiac sympathetic nerve fibers during coronary occlusion. Am J Physiol 226: 603-607.

Uchida Y, Murao S (1974b) Afferent sympathetic nerve fibers originating in the left atrial wall. Am J Physiol 227:753-758.

Uchida Y, Murao S (1974c) Bradykinin-induced excitation of afferent cardiac sympathetic nerve fibers. Jpn Heart J 15:84-91.

Uchida Y, Murao S (1974d) Effects of propranolol on excitation of afferent sympathetic nerve fibers during myocardial ischemia. Jpn Heart J 15:280-288.

Uchida Y, Kamisaka K, Murao S, Ueda H (1974) Mechanosensitivity of afferent cardiac sympathetic nerve fibers. Am J Physiol 226:1088-1093.

Ueda H, Uchida Y, Kamisaka K (1969) Distribution and responses of the cardiac sympathetic receptors to mechanically induced circulatory changes. Jpn Heart J 10: 70-81.

van de Borne P, Montano N, Pagani M, Oren R, Somers VK (1997) Absence of low-frequency variability of sympathetic nerve activity in severe heart failure. Circulation 95:1449-1454.

van Lieshout JJ, Wieling W, Karemaker JM, Eckberg DL (1991) The vasovagal response. Clin Sci 81:575-586.

Vatner SF, Pagani M. (1976) Cardiovascular adjustments to exercise: hemodynamic and mechanisms. Progr Cardiovasc Dis 89:91-107.

Vatner SF, Boettcher DH, Heyndrickx GR, McRitchie RJ (1975) Reduced baroreflex sensitivity with volume loading in conscious dogs. Circ Res 37: 236-242.

Volpe M, Tritto C, De Luca N, Mele AF, Lembo G, Rubattu S, Romano M, De Campora P, Enea I, Ricciardelli B, Trimarco B, Condorelli M (1991) Failure of atrial natriuretic factor to increase with saline load in patients with dilated cardiomyopathy and mild heart failure. J Clin Invest 88:1481-1489.

Von Bezold A, Hirt L (1867) Ueber die physiologischen wirkungen des essigsauren Veratrins. Untersuch Physiol Lab Würzburg 1:73-156.

Wada T, Ono K, Hamada T, Uchida Y, Shimada T, Arita M (1999) Detection of acute cardiac rejection by analysis of heart rate variability in heterotopically transplanted rats. J Heart & Lung Transplant 18:499-509.

Wagner CD, Persson PB (1998) Chaos in the cardiovascular system: an update. Cardiovasc Res 40:257-264.

Wall PD (1985) Future trends in pain research. Philosoph Transactions Royal Soc London B308: 393-401.

Wall PD, Melzack R (1989) Textbook of pain, 2nd ed. Churchill Livingstone, Edinburgh.

Wang W, Zucker IH (1996) Cardiac sympathetic afferent reflex in dogs with congestive heart failure. Am J Physiol 271:R751-R756.

Webb SW, Adgey AA, Pantridge JF (1972) Autonomic disturbance at onset of acute myocardial infarction. Br Med J 3:89-92.

Weidinger F, Hammerle A, Sochor H, Smetana R, Frass M, Glogar D (1986) Role of beta-endorphins in silent myocardial ischemia. Am J Cardiol 58:428-430. ·

Wen ZC, Chen SA, Tai CT, Huang JL, Chang MS (1998) Role of autonomic tone in facilitating spontaneous onset of typical atrial flutter. J Am Coll Cardiol 31:602-607.

White JC (1957) Cardiac pain. Anatomic pathways and physiologic mechanisms. Circulation 16:644-655.

Willis R (1847) The works of William Harvey. Sydenham Society, London.

Woodsworth RS, Sherrington CS (1904) A pseudoaffective reflex and its spinal path. J Physiol (Lond) 31:234-243.

Wolf MM, Varigos GA, Hunt D, Sloman JG (1978) Sinus arrhythmia in acute myocardial infarction. Med J Aust 2:52-53.

Yamamoto Y, Hughson RL, Peterson JC (1991) Autonomic control of heart rate during exercise studied by heart rate variability spectral analysis. J Appl Physiol 71:1136-1142.

Yamamoto WS (1965) Homeostasis, continuity and feedback. In: Yamamoto WS and Brobeck JR (eds): Physiological controls and regulations. WB Saunders Company, Philadelphia and London.

Yanagisawa M, Kurihara H, Kimura S, Tomobe Y, Kobayashi M, Mitsui Y, Yazaki Y, Goro K, Masaki T (1988) A novel potent vasoconstrictor peptide produced by vascular endothelial cells. Nature 332:411-415.

Yo Y, Nagano M, Nagano N, Iiyama K, Higaki J, Mikami H, Ogihara T (1994) Effects of age and hypertension on autonomic nervous regulation during passive head-up tilt. Hypertension 23:I-82 - I-86.

Yotsukura M, Fujii K, Katayama A, Tomono Y, Ando H, Sakata K, Ishihara T, Ishikawa K (1998) Nine-year follow-up study of heart rate variability in patients with Duchenne-type progressive muscular dystrophy. Am Heart J 136:289-296.

Zucker IH, Gilmore JP (1991) Reflex control of the circulation. CRC Press, Boca Raton/Ann Arbor/Boston.

SUBJECT INDEX